WHAT'S
REALLY
WRONG
WITH YOU?

WHAT'S REALLY WRONG WITH YOU?

A REVOLUTIONARY LOOK AT HOW MUSCLES AFFECT YOUR HEALTH

THOMAS GRINER
WITH MAXINE NUNES

Healthy Muscles, LLC

Front Cover: Pablo Picasso's Three Women, 1908
Text Illustrator: Peter Shebell
In-House Editor: David Porrello
Typesetter: Bonnie Freid
Graphic Typesetter: Nuno Faisca

Healthy Muscles, LLC
2323 Bentley, Ste. 303
Los Angeles, CA 90064
www.biopulser.com

Library of Congress Cataloging-in-Publication Data

Griner, Thomas
    What's really wrong with you / by Thomas Griner with Maxine Nunes.
      p. cm.
    Includes bibliographical references and index.
    ISBN 0-89529-658-6
    1. Massage--Therapeutic use.   I. Nunes, Maxine. II. Title.
RM721.G84   1996   95-35289
616.7'4--dc20   CIP

Printed in the United States of America

10 9 8 7

Contents

To the open-minded.

Acknowledgment

I thank Maxine Nunes for her very professional assistance in making the technical information in this book accessible to lay readers.

Preface

The time has come when we can no longer take a submissive role in health care matters. The increasing popularity of alternative health care clearly shows that the experts we entrusted with the care of our bodies have let us down. People are beginning to see that something is rotten in the state of standard health care.

Many medical failures occur because an important area of medicine, with far-reaching effects on health, has been almost totally ignored—muscle. With advanced technology, physiologists have amassed a wealth of information about muscle function, yet doctors (and chiropractors and osteopaths, too) have never investigated and used this knowledge.

Why is it that medical authorities are unable to incorporate important new discoveries about health? One reason is the myth, perpetuated by the American Medical Association, that only their practices are based on scientific proof, while alternative approaches are supported only by anecdotal evidence. The fact is—medicine as it is practiced today is anything but scientific.

In 1989, the United States government formed the Agency for Health Care Policy and Research (AHCPR). Its purpose is to assist in the development and maintenance of national health practice guidelines in order to control runaway medical costs which, if left unchecked, will soon equal the Gross National Product. In 1992, Dr. David Eddy of Duke University, an advisor to the AHCPR, evaluated 21 areas in the field of medicine. Here's what he found: 17 of these areas had little or no scientific validation and existed simply because they were traditional; 99% of the articles in medical journals were scientifically unsound; and 85% of medicine had no scientific basis. It would appear from these findings that the term "medical science" is as much an oxymoron as "military intelligence."

The AHCPR also investigated an area of medical practice particularly relevant to muscle—back problems. According to a study released in December 1994, one of the most costly, unvalidated medical areas is back surgery. This report found that both surgery and physiotherapy were ineffective in treating acute back pain. It stated, "Despite an extensive medical literature on failed back surgery and evidence that repeat surgical procedures for low back problems rarely lead to improved outcome, there are documented examples of patients who have had as many as 20 spine operations." Evidently these "scientific" surgeons consider reports of their failures to be anecdotal.

Muscle physiology, like nutrition, is barely taught in medical schools. Why such glaring omissions? One reason is the considerable influence that pharmaceutical companies have on medical education and practice. One notorious instance of drug company clout involved a therapeutic diet developed at the Johns Hopkins Medical School—a diet that was suppressed because it created "unfair" competition with existing drug approaches.

Drug abuse has thus become another serious medical problem—and I don't mean illegal drugs. Doctors are not only trained to use drugs as quick solutions to medical problems, their prescriptions may also be motivated by drug company perks and inducements. These abuses only surface publicly when famous names like Betty Ford and Elizabeth Taylor become the victims of prescription painkillers. But almost every day, in my practice, I see people who are suffering as a result of medical treatment they have received.

The book you are about to read will help to explain why, for so many conditions, surgery and pharmaceutical treatment are unnecessarily dangerous. It will show you how muscle, which makes up a huge percentage of your body mass, influences every organ and system of your body in profound ways. And it will teach you precisely what goes wrong with your muscles, what kind of trouble this creates, and how your body can be restored to health.

Thomas Griner
Los Angeles, California

Introduction

Sometimes I feel like the boy who said the emperor had no clothes. What I see all too clearly is that doctors do not understand certain conditions that they treat, and often make people sicker with medication and surgery. Alternative approaches such as acupuncture, chiropractic, and various forms of massage may do less harm, but they don't do much good either. One reason for this is a great blind spot—muscle. Most of our body mass is muscle, yet its complex role in health has been almost completely overlooked.

For the past twenty-five years I have been studying muscle. The therapy that grew out of this research has proven to be consistently effective, not only for musculoskeletal problems, but for conditions that are not generally thought of as muscular—allergies, arthritis, asthma, chronic fatigue syndrome, cluster and migraine headaches, and many other disorders.

Once you understand how muscles can affect your health, many of your beliefs about the body will be profoundly altered—as mine were. Let me tell you how my interest in muscle began.

As a child I experienced severe and extremely painful sinus attacks. My father was a chiropractor, and until I was ten years old, the treatments he gave me seemed to help. Then they stopped having any effect at all. By the time I was twelve, any chiropractic adjustment would actually *bring on* a sinus attack. He didn't understand the reason for this, so he stopped working on me, and I learned to endure the attacks.

Because I have always been fascinated with the details of how things work, my first profession was engineering. In the early days of the space program, I did research and testing for the Unmanned Space Program at the Jet Propulsion Laboratory (JPL).

One day while working at JPL, a group of chiropractors asked me, as a research engineering technician, to set up a test to prove the effectiveness of a new technique they had developed. Though the technique itself was much gentler than traditional chiropractic, it was still based on the idea that misaligned bone pinches a nerve, causing a muscle to go into spasm. When I analyzed the tests, I discovered that the the exact opposite was true—the problem actually *began* with muscle spasm. But the chiropractors refused to believe what the evidence showed. And I was left with a fascinating problem: If misaligned bone doesn't cause muscle spasm, what does? No one seemed to know.

I was so intrigued by this question that I enrolled in chiropractic college just to study anatomy and physiology. I took every course offered, but none of them explained muscle spasm.

However, I was able to discover something quite interesting when I experimented on my own muscles. Whenever I found a tight knot, I would begin to probe it with the tips of my fingers. For twenty years I had been playing piano and working in ceramics, so my fingers had developed a certain sensitivity and skill—a kind of knowledge of their own. When I worked on the muscles at the base of my skull with this fingertip technique, an amazing thing happened—my sinuses started draining, and the sinus attacks that had plagued me for my entire life began to disappear.

I started using this fingertip probe on my patients at the school clinic—again with remarkable success. Even before I graduated, I had earned a reputation as someone with a technique that produced dramatic changes when nothing else worked. This technique bore no resemblance at all to any existing type of massage or "deep tissue" work. And although it produced powerful results, I still had no idea why.

After graduation from chiropractic college I was licensed to practice professionally, but I never did. I gave up the license and used the technique I had developed on my own, because it was far more effective in healing the clients who came to me. Yet despite the success of this treatment, the cause of muscle spasm was still a mystery to me. So I went back to the books I had studied in chiropractic school— anatomy, physiology, biochemistry, physical diagnosis, and histology. There is so much information in these volumes that it is impossible to cover it all in just four years of chiro- practic or medical school. But now I knew what I was look- ing for, and I began putting the pieces of the puzzle togeth- er. The information was all there, and I was understanding its implications in a way that no one else had before.

I've written this book to share what I have learned about muscles and their impact on health. Reading it will give you a new and very different understanding of your body, what goes wrong with it, and how it can be healed. But don't expect a simple panacea or a self-help quick-fix. Working with muscle is an art. Like playing the violin, you can read the principles in a matter of hours, but mastery takes a lifetime. This is the first step in understanding the crucial role that muscle plays in your health.

PART ONE

What's *Really* Wrong With You?

If you suffer from back pain, asthma, chronic fatigue, or any other common illness, you are undoubtedly aware of your symptoms. But do you know what *really* causes them?

In the first three chapters of this book, you will learn that the culprit in back pain, asthma, chronic fatigue syndrome and many other common conditions is muscle spasm. If you find this difficult to believe, Chapter 1 may change your mind. It presents case histories of patients with varying conditions, some considered untreatable, whom I have successfully healed.

In Chapter 2, I examine contemporary beliefs about exercise and health which are misleading or untrue. Aerobics and body-building, for instance, are celebrated as keys to health and beauty. Yet, in reality, they are major contributors to muscle spasm and the many illnesses that result from it.

Chapter 3 provides a detailed explanation of the physiology of muscle spasm. It outlines how spasm develops and discusses its impact on the body.

1

A Breakthrough Treatment That Really Works

*T*his book is going to ask a lot of you. First, you're going to have to let go of many beliefs about the body, about fitness, and even about the relationship of mind and body, that may be integral parts of your view of life. Once we've stripped away this foundation of misconceptions, you're going to have to delve into some fairly detailed anatomy and physiology. So before we embark on such a demanding journey together, I want to demonstrate why the information in this book is vital to you.

What I do is based on well-established scientific fact. There is nothing mysterious or mystical about it. There is nothing that must be taken on faith. I don't work with esoteric channels or auras or energies. The knowledge that forms the foundation of this therapy can be found in the same books your doctor studied in medical school. The difference is—according to a 1987 federal inquest into the practices of the American Medical Association—most medical students study muscle physiology for a total of four hours at most. I have been investigating how muscles work for more than twenty-five years.

MUSCLE SPASM

Muscle comprises two-thirds of your body. It has a direct
effect on the nervous system and the circulatory system
and impacts every function of the body—every organ and
every gland. When a muscle is in spasm, it adversely
affects nerves and blood vessels and is a crucial though little understood factor in illness and disease.

Just what is muscle spasm? I will explain it in detail in
Chapter 3. For now, what you need to know is that when
excess lactic acid becomes trapped in a muscle, the muscle
will eventually develop an abnormal, sustained contraction
known as hypertonic spasm. There are other types of spasm,
like a cramp for instance, but hypertonic spasm is what I will
be referring to in this book. Any kind of physical stress,
including too much or too little activity, bumping into furni-
ture, or even slight whiplash, can lead to hypertonic spasm.

It is extremely important to realize that we all have muscle in spasm. But, although spasm causes pain, most of us
are not aware of it. This is because when muscles become
spastic, the body releases its own painkillers called endorphins. Endorphins block the pain of muscle spasm from
reaching your brain. Sometimes spasm is so bad it can cut
off circulation and sensation in nearby nerves. When this
happens, you don't feel pain because the area becomes
numb. But whether you feel pain or not, muscle spasm can
eventually create other physical problems. These include
not only bone, muscle, and joint problems, but a wide range
of conditions, from allergies to blocked arteries.

Most physicians are not aware of the connection
between muscle spasm and illness. They frequently misdi-
agnose patients who have musculoskeletal conditions
such as back, neck, shoulder, and knee pain. As a result,
they often perform surgeries that are unnecessary, ineffective, and damaging. Most of us were raised to place great
trust in medical "science." But how scientific is modern
medicine? In 1989 the United States Agency for Health

Care Policy and Research (AHCPR) was formed to investigate American medical practices. One of this committee's most respected advisors, Dr. David Eddy, found that only one percent of the articles in medical journals were scientifically sound and that *85 percent of medicine had no scientific basis.*

While chiropractors are a lesser evil, they neither understand the origin of muscle spasm, nor have the techniques to alleviate it. They do far less damage than doctors, but they cannot provide a cure for most problems, and eventually aggravate them.

Since we are talking about muscle, you might be wondering at this point whether existing forms of massage can treat spasm. They can't. Superficial massage doesn't even get near the problem, while "deep-tissue" massage, acupressure, and the invasive technique called rolfing make muscles react in a way that actually increases spasm. You may feel better after being treated by one of these methods, but that's only because they have irritated your body enough to produce endorphins and numb your pain.

Before we begin to explore more theoretical and technical information, I want to tell you about some of the clients I've worked with to give you an idea of how effective this treatment is for a wide range of conditions. The names and some personal details have been changed, but the case histories are real. These stories are not the "exceptions." They are typical of the results that have been achieved with thousands of clients during my twenty-five years of practice.

BACK PAIN

According to a study conducted by the Rand Corporation, back pain affects 80 percent of all adults in the United States. Americans spend millions of dollars a year seeking help for this problem, yet available treatments have no lasting effect and will eventually cause even more pain. Surgery, the worst alternative, does nothing to help. In fact, surgery often creates more serious dysfunction, which is complicated even further by the scar tissue it leaves behind.

The Woman Who Tried Everything

For two years, Tracy, a film producer in her early fifties, had suffered from constant, intense lower-back pain. She couldn't sit, stand, walk, or even lie down for any length of time without extreme discomfort.

Before coming to see me, Tracy had tried almost every treatment that promised help, conventional and alternative. Nothing worked. She was treated by several chiropractors with different techniques. They did no good at all. She went to a physician known as the "Ultimate Back Man." He took an MRI, watched her walk, then shook his head and said, "Beats me."

Tracy saw another back expert whose claim to fame was that he could diagnose your problem just by observing the way you walk. He put her through a program of physical therapy, but there was still no change in her condition.

Tracy had spent an enormous amount of money and was becoming very discouraged, but she didn't want to give up. So she traveled to Berkeley, California, to see a famous chiropractor who prescribed *his* therapeutic exercises. They made her back worse. She took yoga classes. They also made her back worse. She had sessions in Alexander technique—a method of treatment that combines physical movement and mental awareness. These sessions did no harm, but they did no good either.

All the effort Tracy made to get help for her lower-back pain had been for nothing. No one had provided any relief. Many had created more pain. By the time she came to me, she really didn't believe that anything could help. When she walked into my office, I could see that one of her hips was protruding more than the other. She had been told that this was caused by a difference in leg length, but it was actually the result of an extremely contracted muscle on one side of her back pulling her torso out of line with her hips.

The muscle on the right side of her spinal column was so hard that when I put her hand on it, she said, "That's not a muscle; that's a bone." When a muscle is that hard, it usually means that the condition has been developing for a long time, even if it has only recently caused pain.

We live in an impatient society, and we want things fixed right away. We're used to solving our physical problems with the scalpel and the pill. But when a condition has taken twenty years to develop, it cannot be gotten rid of overnight. It takes time. I have been releasing Tracy's muscle spasm layer by layer. In a year, we have come a very long way. Her hips are almost even, and she is now virtually pain-free.

"You Need Disc Surgery"

Tracy was lucky. At least she didn't have surgery. Before coming to me, Jack, a physician, had already undergone back surgery three times! His doctors had said the operations were for "herniated" discs, but you'll find out in Chapter 4 why a true herniated disc is so rare as to be almost nonexistent.

When Jack came into my office, he could not walk. A few months earlier, he had been trying to put his dog into his car when he suddenly felt a terrible pain in his back. He couldn't stand or walk, and he had to crawl into the house on his hands and knees.

His doctors took an MRI and told him that he had another herniated disc. They said if he didn't get better, they would have to operate a fourth time. This time Jack was afraid to undergo surgery because the "herniated" disc was in the thoracic area of the spine, which supports the rib cage. As a doctor, he knew that thoracic surgery had a 5- to 10-percent risk of paraplegia. So he lay in bed for a couple of months, unable to walk farther than to the bathroom, until a neighbor suggested that he see me.

I worked on Jack for twenty minutes. When he got up from the table, he was able to walk. He couldn't believe it. He kept saying it was like a miracle. That night, he later told me, he chased his wife all over the bedroom.

I gave him eight more treatments. That was four years ago. He hasn't had any back problems since. "I really didn't need those three surgeries, did I?" he asked me. He certainly didn't.

Can You Trust Your Doctor?

When Peter lost feeling and strength in his arm, his doctor told him he needed surgery immediately. Fortunately, he saw me first.

A year earlier, while skiing, Peter had found himself speeding towards a terrifying choice—drop off a sixty-foot cliff or crash into a retaining wall. He chose the retaining wall and fractured two vertebrae. An orthopedic surgeon gave him a few shots. Peter didn't know what was in these shots. All he knew was that, eventually, the pain disappeared, although his posture remained somewhat stooped.

A few months later, Peter started to get neck pains. One day at the gym, he was lifting some weights over his head when his left hand started to tingle, his fingers went numb, and he lost all strength in his left arm. Over the next few weeks, the left triceps muscle, along the back of his upper arm, began to shrink, as if it were withering away. This really frightened him.

He went to a prominent Los Angeles neurosurgeon who tested his reflexes, then told him that his left triceps was atrophying, or wasting away. "You've got a ruptured disc," the doctor said. "You need an anterior cervical fusion—and any doctor who doesn't know that should give up his license."

An anterior cervical fusion is a surgical procedure performed on the neck portion of the spine. It involves removing the lateral portion of a disc and replacing it with bone, thereby fusing the two adjacent vertebrae. Side effects of this procedure include permanent stiffness in the neck, loss of range of motion, and, for most people, even more pain than before.

Luckily, Peter came to me before subjecting himself to this surgery. The surgeon's examination was so superficial, he had never even touched Peter's muscle. If he had—and if he knew how to interpret what he felt—he would have discovered that, though the muscle was small, it was hard and contracted, not atrophied.

Here's what was *really* wrong with Peter. A nerve in his back was being pinched, not by a disc, but by spastic muscles. Back muscles affected by the ski injury—muscles that run right up into the shoulder—had caused the problems he experienced later with his neck and arm. Drugs had relieved the pain from his original ski injury but they had only covered up the problem.

Peter needed only four treatments to reverse his condition. He no longer has any neck pain; he's recovered the feeling in his arm and fingers; and the size, strength, and reflexes of his triceps have been fully restored. His posture also straightened out, and he regained over an inch in height.

Severe Scoliosis

Peter's height gain was nothing compared with Joe's. Joe, who came to me when he was in his late thirties, was afflicted with severe congenital scoliosis, a curvature of the spine. His was a particularly difficult case because his spine was both curved and twisted. This condition not only affected his appearance and mobility but was also accompanied by chronic pain.

When Joe was in his early teens, doctors put him in a torso cast that extended from his armpits to his pelvis. The cast was almost unbearably uncomfortable and stressed his muscles even more. Doctors told him that if the cast didn't eliminate his pain, they would have to perform surgery. So Joe lied to his doctors, telling them that the cast had worked and his pain was gone. He lied for a good reason. Surgery to correct scoliosis is a grueling ordeal. The surgeon uses an apparatus similar to a ratchet-type car jack to force the spinal curve to straighten. This causes great stress to the back muscles and extremely severe spasm.

When Joe came to me, his progress was slow because he'd had the spinal curvature since birth. The longer a condition goes untreated, the longer it takes to correct. I worked on a thirteen-year-old girl with a similar case of scoliosis, and I was able to straighten her spine in six months. But Joe stayed in treatment for six years. Over that time, there was a dramatic reduction in the distortion of his posture, and he gained several inches in height. Afterward, Joe said, laughing, "Now I look down at people I used to look up to."

ALLERGIES

Allergies are triggered by histamine, and histamine production is affected by the sphenoid sinus located in the center of the head. At the base of the skull is a group of muscles known as the suboccipitals, which have a powerful impact on the sphenoid sinus. They are the key to treating allergies and other conditions involving histamine.

One of my clients, Ruth, had two extremely severe allergies: one to food and the other to paper. She was a customs broker, which involved a great deal of paper work, and for many years she had been allergic to the chemicals with which paper is treated. If she didn't wear special unbleached, white cotton gloves whenever she handled paper, she would break out in a rash. But even the gloves didn't always keep the chemicals from wreaking havoc with her skin.

"My hands don't even look like human hands anymore," she told me the first time she called for an appointment. Her outbreaks would start with a burning red rash. Then she would get boils, which would dry and make the skin of her hands patchy. After that, the skin at the knuckles would split open, sometimes going as deep as the bone, and her hands would swell to three times their normal size. As I worked on her, I could actually see her hands turning from raw red to white. After a few months of treatment, her allergy to paper ceased to be a problem.

Ruth was also allergic to nuts. Several times, while dining out, she would unknowingly eat nuts that had been buried between the layers of a cake or tossed into a salad. Even the tiniest amount would bring on an attack. First, her esophagus would begin to itch. Then her tongue and lips would get hot and her throat would swell up so that she couldn't breathe. On several occasions, she would have died if she had not been rushed to a hospital.

After I treated her, Ruth was understandably afraid to test the results by eating nuts. So for some time we didn't know if the treatment had been successful. Then, one night at a restaurant, she was eating a slice of bread when she suddenly realized that there were nuts in it. Ruth had absolutely no allergic reaction to them at all.

HERPES

The herpes virus causes periodic outbreaks of vesicles, or blisters, which hurt and itch. Attacks can range in intensity from annoying to debilitating. Herpes attacks, like allergy attacks, are triggered by histamine. They can be effectively controlled by massaging the suboccipital muscles at the base of the skull.

Katy, a Los Angeles lawyer in her forties, had been suffering from terrible outbreaks of shingles since she was eighteen. This is a condition in which a herpes virus causes nerve endings, and often the skin, to erupt, producing pain which can be excruciating. Katy had a short series of treatments and hasn't had an outbreak of shingles in a year.

CHRONIC FATIGUE SYNDROME

"I always feel like I'm coming down with the flu." That's how Robin, a political fund raiser, first described her symptoms to me. "I often have a low-grade fever. I'm achy all over, and I get so tired in the middle of the day that I can't stay awake. Sometimes I fall asleep right after breakfast. My brain is in a fog. I can't remember things. My work involves a lot of extemporaneous public speaking, and I've always had a good vocabulary, but now the words just don't come." These are the symptoms of chronic fatigue syndrome.

Friends of Robin with this illness saw their marriages and relationships fall apart. Robin's boyfriend was very supportive, but her career was in jeopardy.

Since doctors have no idea what to do about chronic fatigue syndrome, they often shunt patients from specialist to specialist, and even send them to psychiatrists. Several viruses—among them, the Epstein Barr virus which causes mononucleosis—have been cited as the cause of chronic fatigue. However, these viruses do not cause the problem. They are simply taking advantage of a weakened immune system. Most of us would test positive for some of these viruses, yet never develop any chronic fatigue symptoms.

What is chronic fatigue syndrome? It is an intensified form of hypoglycemia or abnormally low blood sugar. The sphenoid sinus controls not only your histamine level but also your metabolism—and hypoglycemia is a metabolic disturbance. I worked with Robin's suboccipitals to regulate her metabolism, and as a result of this treatment, she's back in high gear again.

DEPRESSION

Anne, a chiropractor, had been severely depressed for most of her adult life, plagued by uncontrollable and unpredictable bouts of crying. She spent long periods of time obsessed with thoughts that kept her locked in a state of emotional pain and profound gloom. Though she was able to function and maintain a small practice, she lived most of her life in anguish.

Anne suffered from two types of depression: agitated and listless. Agitated depression is marked by nervousness and extreme emotional reactions. Listless depression involves feelings of hopelessness, indecisiveness, and an inability to think clearly. In Anne's case, both conditions were the results of chemical imbalances caused by sphenoid sinus irritation.

The agitated depression was caused by excess histamine. Her moods would be darkest when the air was very dry and the pressure was low. This type of weather affects the sphenoid sinus, and can cause extreme emotional reactions in people with sinus problems. That's why, here in California, when the dry, low-pressure Santa Ana winds blow, people tend to have short fuses.

The cause of Anne's listless depression was hypoglycemia. If Anne didn't eat on time her mood would sink. In order to keep her blood sugar up, she had to eat at least six times a day. If she ate sweets for a quick pick-me-up, they would drop her energy level right back down again, plunging her deeper into depression. So she would take food along with her wherever she went.

Through treatment of the suboccipital muscles to reduce histamine and regulate metabolism, Anne's depression has been greatly reduced. She can now eat normally and no longer bursts into tears for no reason at all. When the Santa Ana winds blow, she sometimes experiences a mild change of mood, but it is, she says, nothing compared with the utter despair she suffered before.

ASTHMA

Asthma is a chronic respiratory disease marked by obstructed breathing, chest constriction, and coughing. Though the predisposition to asthma is genetically determined, its symptoms can be controlled by working with muscle. Histamine is one of the factors responsible for asthma attacks. Spasticity in the diaphragm and muscles involved with breathing is another.

Beth was almost sixty and had suffered from asthma all her life. She had been using several different types of medication as well as inhalers to keep the attacks in check. More than once, she had needed emergency inhalation therapy and oxygen to save her life. I started working on her in 1988. During that first year, she stopped taking medication and has not had an attack since.

PARALYSIS

Paralysis, including paraplegia and quadriplegia, usually results from trauma to the central nervous system. Doctors will generally tell you that paralysis occurs because the nerves in the spinal cord have been severed or destroyed. When spinal cord nerves stop functioning, the signal from the brain cannot be transmitted to the muscle. As a result, the muscle atrophies and degenerates. *However, true atrophy exists in only a very small percentage of paralysis cases.*

Most of the time paralysis is caused by a severe contraction of the muscles. This means that a signal from brain to muscle *is* getting through—loud and clear. Instead of a muscle that cannot contract, you have one that is in extreme contraction. This extreme contraction squeezes the blood vessels in the muscle, choking circulation and causing the muscle to shrink in size. That's why doctors mistakenly think it is *atrophied*. But this type of muscle shrinkage is the *opposite* of atrophy; it is *hypotrophy*. The muscle isn't flaccid, it is overly contracted.

Most cases of paralysis involve spasm in its most severe form. Over time, the contraction can be released, and normal function can gradually be restored. When I treat people with paralysis, there is definite, steady, ever-increasing progress. The results may seem slow, but to a paralytic, every increment of change—every tingle where before there was only numbness, every new movement however small—is considered monumental progress. Eventually, modest advances lead to more dramatic change.

The real tragedy is that most paralytics are told that their condition will never improve, and that they have no choice at all but to adjust to their situation. This can be clearly seen in the case of Scott, a young man who refused to accept the hopeless prognosis of his doctors.

Scott, a twenty-two-year-old carpenter with a passion for surfing, was crossing the street one evening when he was hit by a drunk driver going sixty miles-an-hour. Scott went through the car's windshield. He suffered massive head injuries, and his right arm was almost completely severed. When they brought him into the hospital, he was clinically dead. He had no pulse. The doctors were able to save his life, but he was in a coma for three months.

When he regained consciousness and came home from the hospital, the right side of his body was completely paralyzed, his mind was in a fog, and his speech was impaired. A doctor told his brother Robert that some day Scott might be able to turn over and dress himself. This was the best they could expect. The doctors had done an extraordinary job of saving his life. They just didn't have the knowledge or techniques to give him much hope afterwards.

Robert sought alternatives for Scott and found the Feldenkrais technique, a therapy that involves change through awareness. It succeeded in giving Scott greater capabilities within his physical limitations. He learned to stand (with support), to turn over, and to feel more comfortable with his body. He also received some physical therapy and electrical muscle stimulation. However, all of these treatments affected only those muscles that were not paralyzed. They helped him adjust to, but did not change, his paralysis.

The first time I saw Scott he was in a wheelchair. His paralyzed right arm was rigid against his chest, bent at the elbow, his hand useless and curled against his collar bone. His speech was so slow and slurred that it was difficult to understand. Yet because the accident had caused trauma to Scott's brain, he wasn't aware that his speech was impaired.

Almost immediately after the first massage treatment, there was an extraordinary change. Muscle groups which never before had any movement at all, both in Scott's right arm and in his hip area, had begun to come alive. This was a small but very significant change. A few months later, he was able to enroll in a community college. The first semester, he used his wheelchair to get around campus. Then he began to walk, though fairly slowly, with a four-point cane.

Today, Scott uses a single-point cane and can move at a pretty good pace. When he comes to see me, he walks up three flights of stairs to my office instead of taking the elevator. He now has feeling and movement in his fingers, and his right arm has almost completely straightened out. His speech is more fluid and very clear, and his thinking is quicker and more coherent. At school, math had been terribly difficult for him. He could grasp the concepts but couldn't remember them. When I spoke to him recently, he told me that he had received a perfect grade on his last two algebra tests.

A fact not to be overlooked or underestimated about Scott and other paralytics I have worked with is that their own determination and the commitment of their families have been important elements of their success.

AUTOIMMUNE AND METABOLIC DISEASES

One of the most interesting discoveries to have come from working with muscles is that spasm appears to have a direct effect on both autoimmune and metabolic diseases.

In autoimmune diseases (like lupus, rheumatoid arthritis, and multiple sclerosis) the body's immune system attacks its own cells. In metabolic diseases (including diabetes, manic depression, and schizophrenia) there is a disturbance in body chemistry. I have successfully treated many patients with these diseases, and in Chapter 5 we'll discuss how muscle spasm is involved.

Though the number of cases I've dealt with constitutes a limited scientific sample, the results were significant enough to warrant further research.

MANY MORE MUSCLE-RELATED PROBLEMS

There are, in addition to the conditions I have just discussed, numerous physical ailments that are either caused by muscle or can be relieved by treating muscle. These range from bedwetting to blocked arteries, from ulcers to epilepsy. Each of these conditions will be discussed in detail in Part 2, but first let's build a foundation for understanding a completely new system of health treatment.

2

Exposing Some Myths and Misinformation About Health

Wmany ideas and practices, although widely
hen we look back in history, it's easy to see that
accepted in their time, were actually quite
bizarre and even dangerous. During the 19th century, for
instance, physicians still treated fevers with bloodletting—
opening veins to allow demons to escape from the body.
Less than one hundred years ago, in the name of beauty,
women bound themselves into corsets with iron stays that
were so tight, they sometimes damaged internal organs.

We may feel superior to the follies of our ancestors, but
can we see our own? What I want to do now is examine
some contemporary notions about health that most of us
hold unquestioningly—ideas and practices that are not
only wrong, but harmful. I'll cover a wide range of sub-
jects—from aerobics to emotions—and take a look at the
myths and misinformation that keep us from seeing some
basic scientific truths.

EXERCISE

People everywhere are working out because they believe
it's making them healthy and fit. However, as you'll soon

23

see, some of the most widely recommended types of exercise—aerobics, bodybuilding, even yoga—can be quite damaging to the body. These exercises may make you feel good because they force the body to produce endorphins, but later in this section you'll also learn why this endorphin "high" is not a healthy one.

Aerobics

One of the most popular forms of exercise is aerobics—high and low impact aerobics, step aerobics, stairclimbers, stationary bikes, jogging, running, and more.

What's wrong with aerobics? For a start, even the name is misleading. It's based on the idea that when we do "aerobics" our muscles are using oxygen to generate energy. But in reality, the opposite is true. "Aerobics" is predominantly anaerobic. You may be breathing hard, but most of the oxygen *cannot* reach the muscle, and lactic acid is produced.

Another misconception about "aerobics" is that when your heart races it's good for you. It's not. Your heart beats harder because you are in a state of toxicity. The circulatory and respiratory systems automatically respond in this way when something harmful is happening to the body.

One of the main reasons people do "aerobic" exercise is that it's supposed to strengthen the heart. It is true that "aerobics" won't damage the heart itself, because it is the only muscle in the body that can metabolize lactic acid. Unfortunately, your arteries—including the coronary artery to your heart and the pulmonary artery to your lungs—cannot. Lactic acid is irritating to them and may, over time, cause serious problems. That's why you so often hear of joggers needing bypass surgery. It's one of the clues that "aerobic" exercise is harmful, but we are ignoring it.

Bodybuilding

Influenced by new standards of physical attractiveness, both men and women are working out with weights to increase the size and definition of their muscles. But do you know what you are really looking at when you see that "cut" or bulging biceps. It's actually *hypertonic* muscle, muscle in chronic spasm. It is *not* in any way, shape, or form healthy muscle. Bodybuilders are afflicted with muscle so tense, their circulation and nerve function are impaired. And once the muscle is in spasm, whether you stretch it, soak it, or have it massaged, it will stay in spasm. It will remain spastic even when you think you are relaxed. And each time you pump iron, you add to the damage and make the spasm worse. Sooner or later, bodybuilding can lead to back, knee, shoulder and joint injuries, pinched nerves, even serious illnesses.

Poor circulation is another major side effect of bodybuilding. That's why bodybuilders' veins pop to the surface—they can no longer work their way through the hard, permanently contracted muscle. In recent months, two film stars, both known for their muscularity, had to stop work in the middle of production because of pain, swelling, and circulation problems.

Just as a fat person needs extra capillaries to feed his fat, a bodybuilder needs them to feed his muscle. But the bodybuilder is actually in much worse trouble. Fat gives no resistance to capillaries—muscle does. So a bodybuilder is actually putting a greater burden on his heart than someone who is overweight.

Because extreme physical regimens like bodybuilding are so unhealthy, a completely new medical specialty—sports medicine—has been developed in recent years. The question is, how can sports doctors heal a condition if they don't know what really causes it?

Yoga

Most people think of yoga as a harmless, soothing, and beneficial form of exercise, but it really puts an enormous amount of stress on the muscles. That's because the stretching involved in yoga immediately activates a response called the *stretch reflex*, which causes the muscles to contract. As a result, blood circulation becomes strangled and lactic acid accumulates rapidly. By now you know that this will eventually cause spasm.

Why, then, does yoga enable people to increase their range of motion, touch their toes, sit in the lotus position, and appear much more flexible? Because it is their *tendons*—not their muscles—that are being stretched. When you do yoga, the muscle itself actually grows shorter and more tense. If you stop stretching for any length of time, your range of motion will decrease rapidly and you'll see how tight the muscles really are.

While many forms of exercise, even weight training, can be redesigned to become beneficial (you'll see how in Chapter 8), yoga cannot.

"But yoga makes me feel so relaxed," people say. "It gives me such a great sense of well being." Like "aerobics" and bodybuilding, yoga causes enough irritation to produce an endorphin high.

Exercise and Endorphins

Everyone I know who exercises loves the high produced by endorphins—the body's own painkillers. Two hundred times more powerful than morphine, endorphins certainly can make you feel good!

The common belief is that endorphins are nature's reward for exercising. They most emphatically are not. Endorphins are part of your body's fight or flight mechanism. The purpose of endorphins is to enable you to take action when you are injured—to run when you're hurt and an 800-pound gorilla is chasing you. Endorphins are your body's normal response to stress and pain. In order for the body to manufacture endorphins, you have to harm yourself first! The endorphin high that exercisers love is actually an indication of excessive irritation to the body.

In Chapter 1, I said that all of us suffer from some degree of spasticity, whether we know it or not. Endorphins often keep us from feeling the pain of spasm. If you want to know the kind of pain you would feel without endorphins, consider the withdrawal experienced by a heroin addict. When heroin enters the body, it uses the same receptors as endorphins. This causes the body to cease producing endorphins. When the addict stops taking heroin, the agonizing pain of withdrawal is simply the pain of the body without endorphins—the pain that has always been there. That pain is what you would feel right now if your body were not producing endorphins.

Many types of exercise can be addictive, but it is not a "healthy" addiction, as some have called it. Every time you feel that endorphin "high," remember, you are harming your body to get it. Jogging is getting your drugs on the street the hard way. The "fitness" trend is creating a nation of addicts—endorphin junkies who are killing themselves for a fix.

How Much Exercise Is Too Much?

People drastically overestimate the amount of physical stress a body can withstand without adverse reaction. We seem to believe that physical stress always has a positive effect on the body. One fitness guru, whose circulation is so strangled by muscle that his complexion is ash gray, has been telling us for more than forty years, "There's no such thing as too much exercise." That's dangerous misinformation. So is the idea that it is healthy to gradually work up to very strenuous exercise. Both of these concepts are false.

You get two warnings when you have pushed your body too far—fatigue and pain. But fitness "experts" encourage you to ignore them. They advise "running through the pain," and "going beyond the wall," to "have a breakthrough." Doing this is supposed to make you stronger. But what's *really* happening is that you are battering your body into producing enough endorphins to numb the pain. It reminds me of the saying: "Death is nature's way of telling you to slow down." Unfortunately, some people get so numb from excessive exercise, the only message that gets through to them is death.

If Strenuous Exercise is Bad—
Maybe I Shouldn't Exercise at All

Moderation is a dull word. In a world that values speed, excitement, and extremes, it's not a very popular concept. Yet, moderation may well be the most important idea I can impart to you.

So if you're thinking that lying in bed all day might be healthier than performing heavy exercise, I'm afraid that's just as bad. Inactivity also causes lactic acid to accumulate in your muscles, leading to spasm. Your body can endure neither too much activity, nor too much rest.

Moderation in exercise is crucial. The problem is that most people's idea of a moderate workout actually involves extreme exertion. Nevertheless, it is possible to exercise and achieve fitness without killing yourself in the process. I'll tell you how in Chapter 8.

MEDICATION

When something is wrong with our bodies, most of us turn to a doctor. While no one is better at dealing with a life or death physical crisis than a physician, medicine, as it is practiced today, has some severe limitations and drawbacks.

When you take medication—a foreign substance—into your body, there will be side effects, even when they are not immediately noticeable. In certain critical situations, medication may be absolutely necessary. Most of the time, it is not.

You have a whole pharmacy in your body, and many

illnesses are caused when this pharmacy malfunctions. You can take medication, but the chemical imbalance causing the problem can also be regulated by stimulating the nerves through the muscles. In this way, the body can regulate itself, and no foreign substances need be introduced.

Medication is one technique that physicians rely on. The other is surgery.

SURGERY

If your doctor tells you that you need surgery for a "slipped" or "ruptured disc," a "torn rotator cuff," or "carpal tunnel syndrome"—run! I've put quotation marks around these terms for a good reason: They are bogus diagnoses.

Discs don't slip. It's physiological nonsense. And only in the rarest cases do they actually rupture, or tear. In the 1950s, researchers performed postmortems on a group of people who had been diagnosed with "ruptured" discs. Only one-tenth of 1 percent of the sample actually had ruptured discs. But even in the highly unlikely event that a disc does rupture, surgery is probably not the best way to correct the problem.

As for the other diagnoses, today's "torn rotator cuff" was yesterday's "bursitis," and neither term accurately explains the real cause of shoulder pain and what kind of treatment is needed. "Carpal tunnel syndrome" is a fashionable name for a hand problem that doctors do not fully understand and a scalpel cannot cure.

All of these conditions involve muscle spasm and its impact on nerve. Surgery is not the answer. You may feel better shortly after surgery, because the intrusion of a knife into the tissue releases both endorphins and cortisone, producing temporary numbness. However, surgery never addresses the cause of the problem and the source of the pain—muscle spasm. After surgery, the pain almost always returns, and it is usually worse than before.

I had one client who had gone through so much surgery that his friends called him "The Zipper." He had been a professional athlete, which had done a lot of damage to his body. He'd had three operations on his spine, and as a result, those parts of his body that weren't in excruciating pain were completely numb. His left leg dragged behind him, and his right arm hurt so much that when he drove, he had to shift gears with his left hand. Just before he came to me, a team from the prestigious Mayo Clinic in Rochester, Minnesota, told him he needed to have a rod put in his spine. He made a few inquiries and discovered what happened to people who had rods put in their spines. "That's the end of the road," he told me. "They're all in wheelchairs or dead!" It scared him into my office.

When I first saw him, his entire body was as rigid as a wall. He had some of the hardest spasm I have ever seen. The surgeries had left him with massive scar tissue, making it even more difficult to treat him. But in the two years I have been working with him, he has regained feeling in the parts of his body that were numb, and a lot of his pain is gone. His mobility has increased enormously, and he now shifts his car normally—with his right hand. The last thing he needed was more surgery.

Obviously, there are times when surgery is necessary. Physicians are brilliant in certain types of crises. If you have a tumor on your spine, you want a surgeon to remove it. But what happens after surgery, after your healthy tissue has been traumatized by the scalpel? The tumor is gone, but you're left with spasm in the muscles that had surrounded it. This can cause a great deal of long-term pain. Post-surgical massage of muscles can spare a patient years of pain and painkillers.

CHIROPRACTIC

Given what physicians have to offer with drugs and surgery, chiropractic is a less damaging alternative treatment. But a major premise of chiropractic is false. A chiropractor will tell you that misaligned vertebrae have caused muscle spasm, which then pinches nerves and creates pain. But a muscle goes into spasm first, then, eventually, the spasm may pull your vertebrae out of place.

When I was in chiropractic school, students took x-rays before and after performing an adjustment on patients with misaligned vertebrae. The patients would tell us that their symptoms were gone, but when we looked at the x-rays, the misalignment was still there. In some cases, it was even worse than before the treatment. This curious fact, because it contradicted chiropractic theory, was simply ignored by my teachers and colleagues.

A chiropractic adjustment does not straighten your spine. People think the "pop" they hear when a chiropractor works on them is the vertebrae snapping back into place. But this is not the case. Bones don't rub against each other. If they did, it would be catastrophic. A teflon-like cartilage, called hyaline, protects your bones and allows them to glide past each other without wearing out. The sound you hear when a chiropractor "cracks" your back is overly contracted muscle rubbing across the bony surface of the vertebrae.

During a chiropractic manipulation, a chiropractor uses one of several techniques to create traction and stretch the muscle. Stretching a muscle causes a reflex reaction, so the muscle contracts. The chiropractor then jerks the already tight muscle, so it contracts even more. This is very irritating and causes the body to release endorphins, which make you feel better—for a while.

Because it is more conservative than surgery or drugs, chiropractic is less damaging. But in the long run, the irritation and spasm caused by chiropractic treatment will make your condition worse.

ACUPUNCTURE

Acupuncture, which claims to be an almost universal

cure, involves piercing the skin with a needle, sometimes bobbing or twisting it. It also includes moxibustion, a process that heats or burns the skin. All of these techniques can cause muscles under the skin to spasm, and I have seen moxibustion produce spasms the size of a half dollar.

An acupuncture needle can irritate the tissues enough to produce both endorphins, and cortisone, an antihistamine that can produce *temporary* relief of many sinus-related symptoms from depression to a runny nose. This often makes it appear as if acupuncture has "cured" you. The problem is, your body combats *anti*histamine by producing more histamine. After a while, your symptoms will grow worse, and you'll need an increased amount of antihistamine. What acupuncture can and should be used for is anesthesia. It is highly effective and would create far less risk during surgery than chemical anesthetics.

Acupuncture is based on the notion that there are special points on the body which are somehow connected, through invisible channels, to various organs. Yet with all the sophisticated equipment that exists today, with microscopes so powerful we can see atoms, even particles of atoms, no one has ever been able to find a shred of evidence that these mysterious paths of Chinese medicine exist.

Interestingly, however, the acupuncture points do conform to the standard patterns of spasticity. If you put a needle into a non-acupuncture site, the muscle may contract so violently it will pull the needle out of its holder. But if you stick a needle into a spasm, it won't suddenly tighten up. Those chronic spasm sites are the acupuncture points.

People may say, "How can you dismiss a science that is thousands of years old?" But acupuncture is not a science, it's a tradition. Take the mythology away, and the effects of acupuncture are easily explained with modern physiology.

MASSAGE, ACUPRESSURE, ROLFING, AND REFLEXOLOGY

Standard massage can be temporarily soothing, but it reaches only the surface muscles and doesn't get near the deep-seated muscles which are in spasm. You'll feel better right after a massage, but within hours, the tension will return.

Many types of massage are referred to as "deep-tissue" massage, but that is totally misleading. These techniques never even reach the deeper muscles. Whenever you press on a muscle, the superficial muscles immediately tense up, preventing you from going any deeper. People often ask me if I do deep-tissue massage, and I say, "Yes. *Eventually*," because you have to work with the layers on top before they will allow you to go deeper.

Acupressure and shiatsu, its heaviest form, are very irritating to the system. The muscles are pressed on with such force, they react by tensing up.

Rolfing is an extreme form of heavy massage. It is based on a theory that has no physiologic basis whatsoever—that there are adhesions (scar-like tissue) on structures called fascia which surround the muscles. The knots rolfers feel are not "adhesions" but spastic muscle, which they try to smash with great force as if it were scar tissue. Rolfing exerts an excruciating pressure on the muscle, which can only react by tightening.

Reflexology, a type of foot massage, is another treatment based on an idea with no basis in physiology. Reflexologists feel hard knots in the feet and call them "crystallizations," which they believe are, in some mysterious way, connected to various organs in the body. What are these tiny knots that can be felt in the feet? You guessed it. Spasm.

Massage treatments that irritate the body may make you feel better for a while because of the endorphins they produce.

HOT BATHS AND SAUNAS

Many people take a hot bath or sauna after a workout or when they want to unwind. They think that they're helping their muscles to relax. In fact, just the opposite is happening. Heat as well as cold causes thermal shock. Your body has an elaborate mechanism to maintain your set temperature. When you do things to offset it, you irritate the body. When you sit in a hot tub, cooking like a lobster, your muscles do not relax—they draw tighter and tighter.

Contrary to popular belief, heat does *not* improve circulation. It dilates the capillaries and slows the flow of blood. When you sit in a hot tub and your skin turns red, it's not because your blood is coursing through you. It's because the blood has slowed down so much that it has accumulated in your blood vessels. Occasionally, you hear of someone who has had a heart attack while drinking alcohol in a hot tub. This happens because the combination of alcohol and heat dilates the blood vessels to such an extent that there is not enough blood pressure to pump blood back to the heart.

Saunas can be bad for circulation too. A PBS television program followed three men through a sauna. Before they went in, their blood pressure readings were normal—120 over 80. In fifteen minutes, their pressures rose to 190 over 150. After the sauna, they jumped into a cold stream—thermal shock on top of thermal shock. Their pressure readings rose to 300 over 250. Perhaps these men believed that subjecting themselves to such extreme stress would make them strong. It didn't. But it could have led to a heart attack or stroke.

Why do you feel so good after a hot bath or a sauna? First, in response to all the irritation, your body starts producing endorphins. Second, heat acts as an analgesic, or painkiller, on the nerve endings. This produces a feeling of well-being, despite the fact that muscles are going into spasm.

MIND OVER MATTER

There seems to be a widespread idea that if you are some-how strong enough, or aware enough, or if you meditate enough, you can control your body with your mind. There are people who believe that if they develop their "con-sciousness" they will be able to control their unconscious physical functions and prevent or cure their own illnesses. This expectation is extremely misguided. I have worked on Buddhist lamas and Hindu gurus, very wise and holy men who have devoted their lives to meditation and spiritual pursuits. They suffer from the same ailments as the rest of us, and they require the same physical treatment to heal them.

People who are fascinated by Eastern mysticism love to hear stories about yogis in caves who can stop their hearts from beating, or men who pierce their flesh with knives and never bleed. They believe that with enough dedication, anyone can develop these extraordinary skills. But this is simply not so. Like a photographic memory, these abilities can only be developed if you are born with them. The rest of us can sit in a cave and meditate for fifty years, and we still won't have the power to stop our hearts at will or make our blood clot. What we will have is spasm—from sitting for too long in the lotus position.

Another approach to attaining mind over matter is biofeedback. This technique uses a machine to monitor brain waves or muscle activity, and is supposed to help control certain bodily functions. Several years ago, biofeed-back was hailed as the great new hope for a host of condi-tions, from high blood pressure to migraine headaches. What happened to this miracle cure? For approximately 15 percent of the people who tried biofeedback, it worked very well. For another 15 percent, it had absolutely no effect at all. For the remaining 70 percent, the influence was too mild to be significant.

The statistics break down exactly the same way for

hypnosis. At one time it was thought that hypnosis might replace anesthesia as an artificially induced sleep. Like biofeedback, hypnosis was able to control pain for about 15 percent of the people who tried it. However, it had absolutely no effect on another 15 percent of people, and had partial but inadequate success with the remaining 70 percent.

So you can see, for 85 percent of us, the notion that we can control our bodies with our minds is unrealistic.

EMOTIONAL STRESS AND MUSCLE

Just mention muscle tension and the first thing people think of is emotional stress. The belief that emotional upset causes muscle tension is firmly entrenched—but physiologically impossible. Emotions have a powerful influence on many functions of the body—but virtually none on our muscles.

Most of us are like my client Christine, who came in one day with an acute pain in her shoulder. She was convinced it was the direct result of emotional stress. "I was at a very rough business meeting," she said, "and I could feel my muscles knotting up until they were aching." I treated her, not only to relieve the pain, but to reduce some of her chronic muscle spasm. About a week later, she had another meeting. It was even more stressful emotionally—but there was no pain in her shoulder because we had gotten rid of some deep spasm. Emotions may *trigger* muscle problems—but the cause always has its roots in existing physical spasm.

There are two popular images that reinforce the myth of emotionally induced muscle tension. One is that of a deer "frozen" in the headlights of a car. The deer's reaction, however, is not caused by muscular tension. It is an instinctive reflex, a "statue act," to help the deer hide from predators by blending into the background. Unfortunately for the deer, this ancient instinct just doesn't work with cars.

The other image is of someone in panic "paralyzed

with fear." But when you see any news story about people in panic, they aren't frozen in place, they're stampeding like scared cattle. Their muscles are working just fine. If people "freeze" in stressful situations, it is because of mental confusion or conflict, not physiological muscle lock-up. The fight or flight mechanism insures that emotional disturbance does not interfere with muscles. Otherwise, man would have been driven to extinction like the dodo bird.

The idea that emotions have an impact on muscle was taken to its extreme about sixty years ago by psychologist Wilhelm Reich. He believed that we develop a "muscular armor" in response to the emotional pain of childhood. This theory gave rise to a multitude of therapies based on the premise that an emotional memory is somehow trapped inside the muscle—that if you've got knots in your shoulder, it's because your mother yelled at you thirty-five years ago; if you have migraine headaches, it's because your repressed emotions are getting back at you. I even saw one book that claimed lower back problems were caused by money worries!

The only time there is a connection between emotion and muscle spasm is when the *physical* event causing the spasm had an emotional element to it. I'll give you an example. A few years ago a woman came to me suffering from severe spasm in her arms and shoulders. When I worked on her, she burst into tears while remembering an incident from her childhood. When she was three years old, her brother threw her over the balcony of their second floor apartment. She was hanging on for dear life while he tried to pry her fingers from the railing. She hung there, crying and screaming, for several minutes until her mother finally came out and rescued her. When I worked on her, the memory came back and she cried like a little girl, because the physical stress in her arm muscles had been accompanied by a strong emotion. This direct link between emotion and muscle occurs only when physical and emotional traumas happen *simultaneously*.

The Physiological Facts

Emotions *do* have an influence on many bodily functions.

Every emotional response has a physiological reaction. This occurs primarily in a part of the brain called the *limbic system*, the emotional center of the brain. A part of the limbic system called the *amygdala* is responsible for our immediate reactions. The amygdala causes us to cry when we're sad, blush when we're embarrassed, and smile when we're happy.

Another part of the brain, the *hippocampus*, is involved in learning and memory. The limbic portion of the hippocampus is devoted to emotional memory. It's what gives us a feeling of déjà vu when we experience a familiar sight, sound, taste, odor, or touch. It's what triggered the tears of the woman who was thrown off a balcony as a little girl.

The limbic system is located near the *hypothalamus*, which is the control center of the *autonomic nervous system*. This is the part of the brain that directs involuntary functions such as heart rate, digestion, and glandular activity. The nerve routes that connect the hypothalamus and the emotional limbic system are short and direct. Because of this link, emotions have a direct impact on the autonomic nervous system. That's why emotions can have a huge impact on your health.

Table 2.1 will show you the great number of bodily functions that are controlled by the autonomic nervous system and, therefore, influenced by emotion. But there are only two muscle functions that emotions affect—shivering and quivering.

All other skeletal muscle function is controlled by the cerebrum and cerebellum. These two parts of the brain are located far from—and have absolutely no connection to—the emotional limbic system. This makes it impossible for emotions to have any direct effect on muscles.

The primary cause of muscle tension is physical—not emotional—stress. Every time you bump your head, knock your leg against the corner of a table, or even cross your legs for too long, your muscles are affected more than when you have a domestic spat or a problem at work.

However, while emotions do not make for tense muscles, the condition of your muscles can determine your emotions. If your muscles are irritable, you will be too. If they're tight, you'll be uptight. Your body does not reflect your emotions. Your emotions reflect your body.

FACT VERSUS FICTION

Sometimes it's painful to replace fiction (B.S.) with fact (reality). But once you do, you have a valid base on which to reach some solid conclusions. In this chapter, a whole herd of sacred cows needed to be slaughtered. So, now, let's get onto the beef using the facts of science to explain how good muscle actually goes bad.

Table 2.1. Emotions and the Body

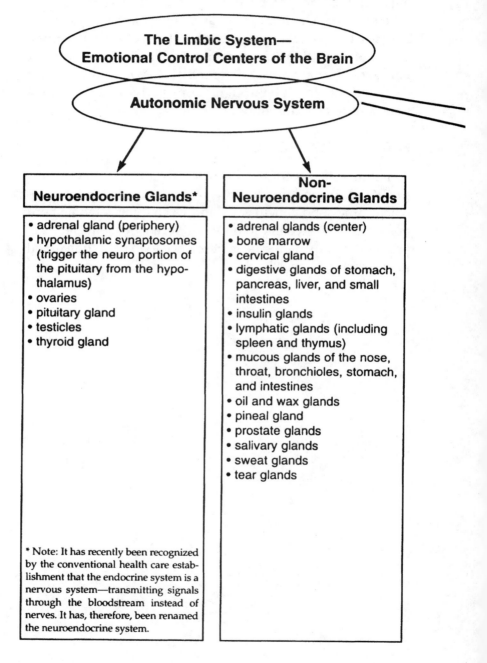

**The Limbic System—
Emotional Control Centers of the Brain**

Autonomic Nervous System

Neuroendocrine Glands*	Non-Neuroendocrine Glands
• adrenal gland (periphery) • hypothalamic synaptosomes (trigger the neuro portion of the pituitary from the hypo-thalamus) • ovaries • pituitary gland • testicles • thyroid gland	• adrenal glands (center) • bone marrow • cervical gland • digestive glands of stomach, pancreas, liver, and small intestines • insulin glands • lymphatic glands (including spleen and thymus) • mucous glands of the nose, throat, bronchioles, stomach, and intestines • oil and wax glands • pineal gland • prostate glands • salivary glands • sweat glands • tear glands

* Note: It has recently been recognized by the conventional health care establishment that the endocrine system is a nervous system—transmitting signals through the bloodstream instead of nerves. It has, therefore, been renamed the neuroendocrine system.

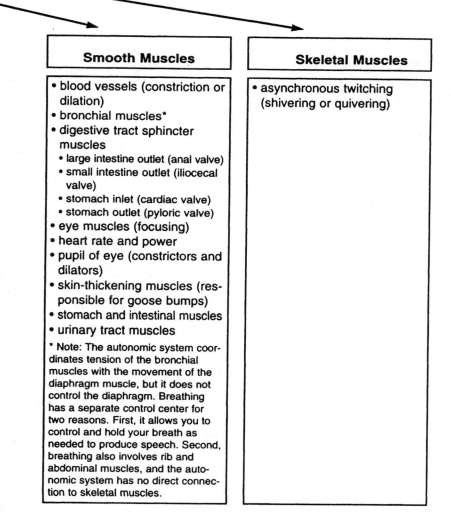

Smooth Muscles	Skeletal Muscles

• blood vessels (constriction or dilation)
• bronchial muscles*
• digestive tract sphincter muscles
  • large intestine outlet (anal valve)
  • small intestine outlet (iliocecal valve)
  • stomach inlet (cardiac valve)
  • stomach outlet (pyloric valve)
• eye muscles (focusing)
• heart rate and power
• pupil of eye (constrictors and dilators)
• skin-thickening muscles (responsible for goose bumps)
• stomach and intestinal muscles
• urinary tract muscles
 	
* Note: The autonomic system coordinates tension of the bronchial muscles with the movement of the diaphragm muscle, but it does not control the diaphragm. Breathing has a separate control center for two reasons. First, it allows you to control and hold your breath as needed to produce speech. Second, breathing also involves rib and abdominal muscles, and the autonomic system has no direct connection to skeletal muscles.
	• asynchronous twitching (shivering or quivering)

3
Spasm—How Good Muscles Go Bad

Hypertonic Spasm—The excessive, insidious, permanent contraction of a muscle caused by an accumulation of concentrated lactic acid.

Everything from pop culture to language itself conspires to give muscle a kind of second-class status. Muscle is the dumb jock, the gangster's body guard, the beefcake, and the brute. Even doctors seem to have been influenced more by movies than muscle physiology. Muscle is not considered important enough to be taught in-depth in medical schools. There its role in overall health and body function is drastically underestimated. Moreover, a critical type of muscle dysfunction—spasm— is not understood by doctors.

There are many types of muscle spasm, from cramps to tics, but the spasm we are concerned with here is distinctly different from these. Technically, it is known as *hypertonus*—excess muscle tone caused by an accumulation of concentrated lactic acid in the muscle. This type of spasm is permanent unless treated. But until symptoms begin to appear, we rarely feel pain from or have any awareness of this type of spasm. This is why I call it "insidious" spasm.

INSIDIOUS SPASM

Insidious spasm exists in everyone to some degree—even in babies. I've often heard people say, "Babies can't hurt themselves; they're made out of rubber." But babies are made of exactly the same stuff adults are. If you palpate a baby's muscles, you will become aware of the significant amount of spasticity already there.

In fact, a baby's muscles build up lactic acid even before birth. The muscular system of a fetus is completely formed by the fifth month of gestation. From then on, because there is so little movement in the womb, lactic acid begins to accumulate. That's why at birth, an infant's arms and legs are bent, and the tiny fists and toes are often curled. The birth trauma itself causes still more stress to the muscles.

It's hard for people to accept that newborns have spasm. Most of us want to believe that we start out with a perfectly designed system and mess it up ourselves as we go through life. But humans did not spring up whole in finished and impeccable form. Rather, like all species, we evolved by adapting to what was needed. And we are still adapting. As a result, the body has a few built-in glitches. One of them is insidious spasm.

Two factors that are crucial to understanding insidious spasm were not known until after World War II. One was the discovery of endorphins—the body's own painkillers. The other involved new details about muscle function, which appeared in the 1960s in the *Textbook of Medical Physiology* by Arthur C. Guyton, a standard text in medical and chiropractic schools. Unfortunately, because the significance of this information was not recognized, some of it disappeared from later editions. Yet, even if you had read the sixties edition of Guyton from cover to cover, the phenomenon of spasm may not have been apparent because the relevant facts were scattered throughout its pages like the pieces of a puzzle. Only because I was specifically searching for the etiology, or cause, of spasm was I able to see the whole picture.

By the time you have finished this chapter, you'll have learned some key facts about muscle that your doctor and chiropractor probably don't know. We'll cover enough basic muscle physiology for you to understand exactly what kind of muscle becomes spastic and why. You'll also begin to see the wide-reaching effects muscle can have on your health.

MUSCLE

You are mostly muscle. Your body has more muscle than any other type of tissue. In the average person, about two-thirds of body mass is muscle—tissue rich with blood vessels and nerves, influencing every organ and every system of the body.

There are three types of muscle: cardiac, smooth, and skeletal. They have different functions and different structures. They also differ in the way they are affected by lactic acid—a by-product of muscle activity and the cause of spasm.

Cardiac Muscle

Cardiac muscle is found only in the heart. It is made up of thick, spiral bands which continuously contract and relax in order to pump blood through your body. When blood sugar is low, the heart is able to use lactic acid for fuel. It is the only muscle in the body that can do this because it is rich in both oxygen and the necessary enzymes. For this reason, the heart itself cannot become spastic.

Smooth Muscle

The action of smooth muscle is involuntary. It is controlled by the autonomic nervous system, which is in charge of your body's unconscious functions. Smooth muscle is found in the intestines, the lungs, the uterus, the iris of the eye, and many other internal organs. It also comprises the walls of your blood vessels, including your arteries.

The arteries do not produce a great deal of lactic acid themselves, but they must carry the lactic acid produced by other muscles.

When spasm occurs in an artery, it begins to degenerate and shed cells, forming tiny bumps on the artery walls. These bumps attract cholesterol, which creates the plaque that causes blockage and can lead to a heart attack. Concentrated lactic acid in the blood can also cause clotting in the veins. This is what causes hemorrhoids, which are clots in the veins of the anal sphincter muscle, and thrombophlebitis, a clot in a vein of the calf.

Skeletal Muscle

The third type of muscle—which comprises 99 percent of the body's muscle mass—is skeletal muscle.

All skeletal muscles have tendons which attach the muscle to bone and also act as shock absorbers.

Skeletal muscles are made up of two distinct types of fibers: dark, or slow-twitch fibers; and white, or fast-twitch fibers. Recognizing the differences between them is important in understanding metabolism and exercise, and you'll learn more about these differences in Chapter 8.

What's most important for you to know right now is that there are two types of skeletal muscle: flat and round. This is a crucial distinction because while round skeletal muscles can become spastic, flat skeletal muscles, except at their attachments to bone, cannot.

Flat skeletal muscles and their tendons are arranged in

sheets, which attach to the bone in a line, as shown in Figure 3.1. When a flat muscle contracts, the tension is distributed evenly in a plane. This conformation of muscle, cannot trap lactic acid, so these muscles are not subject to insidious spasm. Even if the flat muscle has many layers and is very thick, it will not become spastic. The *latissimus dorsi* of the back and the *gluteus maximus* of the buttocks are examples of flat muscles.

Round muscles and their tendons attach to bone between two points, as shown in Figure 3.1. In order for tension to be evenly balanced around the line between the two points, all muscle fibers which contract simultaneously must be arranged in concentric cylinders with that line at their center. When round muscle contracts, it closes like a fist around the blood vessels, trapping lactic acid. The *biceps* and *brachialis* muscles of the arm are primarily composed of round muscle, while groups like the *deltoid* of the shoulder and *pectoralis major* of the chest are made up of both flat and round sections.

All skeletal muscles—flat and round—and their tendons can become spastic at their *attachments*. This is because muscle attachments curve inward just before they attach to the bone (as in Figure 3.2) allowing lactic acid to become trapped.

You may have learned in school that skeletal muscle is sometimes called "voluntary" muscle. This is not entirely accurate because skeletal muscles are under both conscious and unconscious control. This fact is a key to understanding muscle tone—the next piece of our puzzle.

MUSCLE TONE

We tend to think of muscle tone as it relates to beauty and appearance. But what exactly is muscle tone? It is the amount of contraction that remains when a muscle is relaxed. Muscle tone has a very important purpose: It holds your skeleton in place when you are at rest. But most

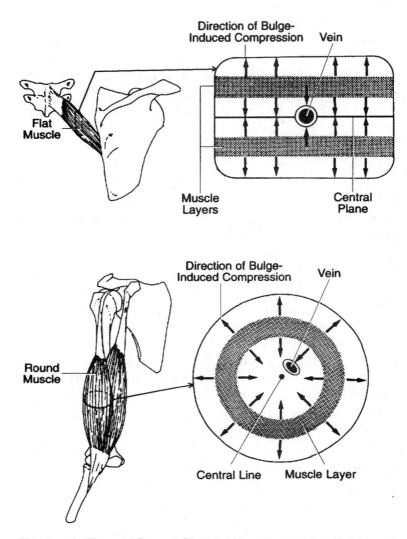

Figure 3.1. Flat and Round Skeletal Muscle. A contracting muscle bulges, as when you flex your biceps. This bulging produces compressive force on the adjacent tissues. When a flat muscle contracts, compression is distributed evenly in a plane. The blood vessels remain open, lactic acid does not become trapped, and the muscle does not become spastic. A round muscle attaches to bone between two points. When the muscle contracts, it closes like a fist around the blood vessels, trapping lactic acid and eventually causing spasm.

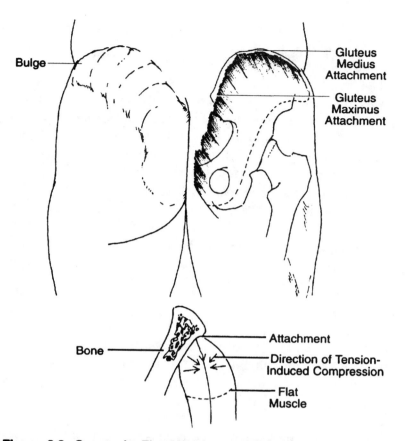

Figure 3.2. Spasm In Flat Muscle Attachments. Generally, flat muscle, because of its shape, is not susceptible to spasm. However, at its attachment to bone, flat muscle is rounded and can become spastic. The dark areas show the spasm that occurs along the attachments of the gluteus maximus and gluteus medius. The bulge along the muscle attachments is typical of dancers and other athletes.

health care providers do not understand this. They believe that ligaments hold the body in place. However, this is physiologically impossible. Ligaments are bands of tissue that connect the bones to each other. The ligaments of most joints are slack. They become taught only when you go beyond your normal range of motion. Ligaments are, in fact, a backup system for your muscles. Their sole purpose is to keep you from going further out of joint only *after* a dislocation has taken place.

Unlike muscles and tendons, ligaments cannot stretch. The layers of tissue in a ligament are crisscrossed in such a way that they lose all elasticity. This pattern is shown in Figure 3.3. (The vocal ligaments and the ligamenta flava— which protects the spinal chord—are exceptions.) If ligaments were tight enough to hold your joints in place, you would not be able to move!

Muscle tone alone maintains your posture. For this reason, no healthy muscle is ever completely slack. If your muscles were ever to relax totally, you would go right out of joint. In order to maintain tone, the brain directs constant *involuntary* muscle activity. Like the heart, our muscles are always at work, twenty-four hours a day, even when we are asleep.

How The Brain Maintains Muscle Tone

A muscle moves in only two ways: It either contracts or relaxes. For movement to occur, the brain must send an impulse through the nerves, down the spinal cord, and to the muscle. When movement of muscle is conscious, the part of the brain known as the *cerebrum* gives the command. When movement of muscle is unconscious, the *cerebellum* is in charge.

The maintenance of muscle tone involves unconscious muscle contraction and is also controlled by the cerebellum. But how does the cerebellum know what instructions to give to the muscles? Muscles have feedback nerves, which are like reporters on the front lines. They're out there where the action is, sending information back to the brain. If the signal from the feedback nerves is weak, the cerebellum tells the muscles to tighten up. If the signal is strong, the cerebellum tells the muscles to relax.

These feedback nerves (as well as the nerves that control the stretch reflex) are located in a part of the muscle called the spindle.

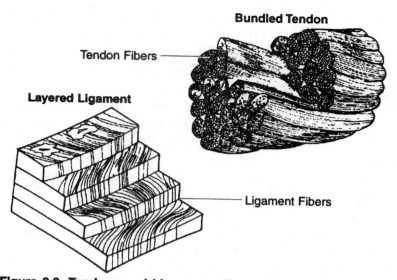

Figure 3.3. Tendons and Ligaments. The parallel conformation of collagen fibers in tendons retain elasticity like little coiled springs. The crisscrossed pattern of collagen fibers in ligaments inhibits elasticity.

THE MUSCLE SPINDLE

Inside the muscle is a complicated structure called a muscle spindle, shown in Figure 3.4. It gets its name from the membrane that encloses it, which is tapered on the ends like a spindle. Unfortunately, this membrane, intended for protection, also acts as an accumulating repository for lactic acid generated by the surrounding forest of working muscle fibers. The spindle membrane encloses two types of delicate muscle fibers—one for muscle tone, the other for stretch-reflex control.

The stretch reflex is what causes a muscle to automatically tighten when you stretch it. It also causes the knee-jerk response that occurs when the tendon next to the knee cap is stretched by a light tap. (The stretch reflex will have critical importance in Chapter 7, when we discuss how to correct excess muscle tone.)

The muscle fiber associated with stretch reflex is called

a bag fiber because its nuclei are lumped together in a central bag. The ends of the bag fiber are attached to two different points on a working muscle fiber, so that information about the length of the working muscle fiber is physically transferred into the spindle.

The muscle fiber involved with muscle tone is called a chain fiber because its nuclei are strung end-to-end in a slender line. The ends of the chain fiber are attached to two different points on the bag fiber, so that information about both the working muscle fiber and the bag muscle fiber are physically transferred into the chain muscle fiber.

Feedback nerves, called flower-spray nerves because of their resemblance to flowers, are attached near the ends of the bag and chain fibers. Most of the flower-spray nerves inform the cerebellum about the state of the muscle. The cerebellum then sets the tone for the working muscle. When the lactic acid trapped in the spindle membrane sickens these nerves, they send a weakened signal to the cerebellum, which then commands the muscle to tighten. And that's the start of muscle spasm.

A small number of flower-spray nerves act as stretch-reflex feedback nerves. As you might expect, they are also sickened by lactic acid, so that wherever muscle tone is excessive, the stretch-reflex response is heightened. This can't cause problems the way excess muscle tone can—but an exaggerated knee-jerk response is usually good for a laugh.

Both the bag and the chain fibers are connected to activate the working muscle fibers through anulospiral nerves which spiral around the middle portion of the bag and chain fibers.

What a complicated mess! With so many cooks, no wonder the broth is so easily spoiled. Rube Goldberg would be envious.

A muscle at rest may appear static, but it is working constantly to maintain tone and to keep the body in proper posture. These generally unrecognized facts are key elements in

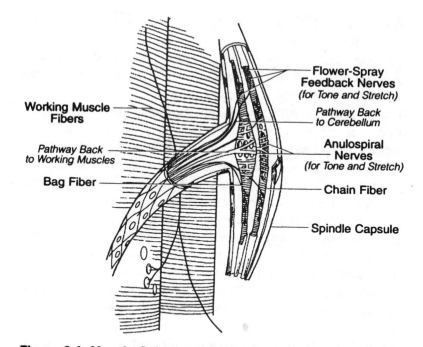

Figure 3.4. Muscle Spindle and Feedback Nerves. The spindle houses the nerves that maintain the muscle tone and elasticity. The flower-spray feedback nerves attach near the ends of the bag and chain fibers and communicate with the cerebellum, which sets the level of muscle tone and elasticity. The anulospiral nerves attach at the middle of the fibers, and communicate directly with the working muscle.

understanding spasm. You'll have the whole picture when you see how feedback nerves are affected by lactic acid.

LACTIC ACID

Lactic acid is our villain—the cause of hypertonic spasm.

Lactic acid is produced when an animal cell metabolizes sugar anaerobically—without using oxygen. Whenever your muscles are at work—and that's all the time—they produce lactic acid. The harder and more sustained the muscle activity, the greater the output of lactic acid.

Lactic acid was first discovered in milk, where it is produced when *lactobacillus acidophilus* bacteria metabolize the milk sugar lactose (hence the name lactic acid).

The lactic acid in milk products is so diluted, it's harmless to you. But the lactic acid your own body manufactures can cause problems. Lactic acid can cause your blood to clot, just as it causes milk to thicken and ferment in the production of sour cream and yogurt. Also, in high concentrations, lactic acid can be so toxic to tissue that when it is dropped on living cells in a test tube, the cells will sizzle and burn.

When a muscle contracts and metabolizes glucose for energy, it first produces pyruvic acid. Pyruvic acid can be cleanly burned if there is enough oxygen in the muscle. If there is not enough oxygen in the muscle, pyruvic acid turns into lactic acid. There are two reasons a muscle creates lactic acid. First, if the muscle contracts strongly enough, it can shut off its own blood supply and, therefore, its supply of oxygen. And second, your fast-twitch muscle fibers can only metabolize glucose anaerobically. So, even when you are at rest, about 20 percent of muscle metabolism produces lactic acid. The percentage rapidly increases as you move.

While skeletal muscles produce the greatest quantity of lactic acid in the body, they do not have enough oxygen and/or enzymes to metabolize it. Only two organs are always supplied with an adequate amount of oxygen and enzymes to effectively metabolize lactic acid. They are the heart and the liver. The heart will metabolize lactic acid only when it needs it for energy. The remaining lactic acid produced by the body must be processed by the liver. The liver uses only the lactic acid it needs for energy, converts the rest into glucose, and sends the glucose back through the bloodstream to be used by the tissues as fresh fuel.

The body knows how toxic lactic acid is. That's why the veins from the anal sphincter—which is almost always contracted and produces enormous amounts of lactic acid—are routed directly to the liver to prevent dangerous levels of lactic acid in the bloodstream.

When you exercise, lactic acid forces your heart rate up

and makes you breathe hard because you need more oxy-gen—not just for your muscles, which cannot take in enough oxygen to metabolize lactic acid during sustained exercise—but also for your liver.

If the lactic acid can be flushed out of the muscle and carried in the bloodstream to the liver, it will be metabo-lized. However, under certain circumstances, lactic acid becomes trapped in the muscle, where it grows more and more concentrated. This is the beginning of spasm.

HOW SPASM DEVELOPS

As you now know, when a round muscle contracts, it squeezes tightly around its own blood vessels and com-presses them. This causes a significant decrease in the flow of blood. If the contraction is particularly strong, blood flow may be totally stopped. This means that during a contrac-tion, the lactic acid being produced cannot leave the muscle.

From the moment a muscle contracts, lactic acid starts to accumulate. When it becomes concentrated enough to be toxic, it begins to make trouble.

During prolonged exertion, concentrated lactic acid col-lects in the muscle spindles and begins to affect the feedback nerves. Their signals grow weaker and weaker, and the cere-bellum interprets this to mean that the muscle is relaxing. So it commands the muscle to tighten up. Tightening an already tight muscle produces and traps still more lactic acid, further weakening the signal from the feedback nerves. The cerebel-lum then makes the muscle tighten up even more. Thus begins a vicious cycle of self-sustaining spasm that, over time, intensifies and grows larger.

WHY YOU MAY NOT FEEL PAIN
FROM INSIDIOUS SPASM

There are two reasons you may not feel pain from insidious spasm. The first is that your deeper muscles are insensate, that is, they do not have pain nerves. Any pain that you feel from spasm is a result of irritation being transmitted to the surface muscles. What turns the surface pain off is the release of endorphins, which we discussed briefly in Chapter 2. Now let's take a closer look at exactly how these natural painkillers are created by the body and how they can affect it.

HOW THE BODY RELEASES ENDORPHINS

When the body is irritated, the pituitary gland manufactures endorphins from a large molecule called a *betalipoprotein*. The endorphins then travel from the pituitary to receptors in a part of the brain called the *amygdala*, where they block pain transmission.

The word endorphin means "internal morphine." Its effects were first observed during World War II, when doctors noticed that soldiers suffering from severe injuries often felt no pain. These soldiers were too lucid to be in shock, yet amazingly, they were able to undergo surgery without any anesthesia. The cause of this phenomenon, called the "pain gate," remained a mystery for decades.

About twenty-five years ago, scientists used radioactive tags to study how morphine functions in the body. They discovered that the drug always went to specific receptor sites in the brain. Here was another mystery: Why did the brain have receptor sites for morphine, a foreign substance? The scientists reasoned that there must be some chemical produced by the body that is similar to morphine, and for which these receptors had been developed.

During the mid-1970s, scientists discovered endorphins. Endorphins used the same receptor sites as morphine—and matched those sites perfectly, where morphine did not. That's why endorphins are two hundred times more powerful than morphine in blocking pain transmission. It's also the reason endorphins do not produce the adverse side effects that morphine does.

While doctors during World War II assumed that only severe trauma brought about the "pain gate," scientists later found that a wide range of irritation—from acupuncture to aspirin—could cause the production of endorphins. Even the ingestion of sugar by people who are sugar sensitive can trigger endorphins.

Lactic acid, which is highly irritating, also causes the pituitary to release endorphins. Endorphins numb the pain that lactic acid would otherwise cause. That's why the more spasm you have, the less likely you are to feel it—until it causes something in the body to go wrong.

Have you ever had pain that seemed to appear out of nowhere? You probably dismissed it with an excuse like "I slept wrong," or "I get this way every six months, but it always goes away." What *really* happens is that spastic muscle you never felt before touches other organs or nerves not yet numbed by endorphins. This can occur because you moved at an odd angle or because the spasm has grown into a new area. But long before you felt pain, the spasm was there. And it will remain even after the pain disappears. Time does not heal all wounds—only your awareness of them.

MUSCLE RESERVE

The more your muscles become dysfunctional with spasm, the more they begin to use up the healthy muscle your body holds in reserve.

You've probably heard it said that 80 percent of our brain remains unused. It's commonly believed that this untapped capacity implies some extraordinary human potential. What most people don't realize is that this impressive amount of unused tissue exists only in the average 18-year-old. It is actually reserve tissue, whose purpose is to replace, as needed, cells which may die or become dysfunctional.

This is also true for muscles. Most of us will begin to

exhaust our muscle reserve between fifty and fifty-five. That's why, at about that age, people begin to notice stiffness and pain in their joints, as well as a decrease in their range of motion, speed, and physical stamina.

Reducing your supply of reserve tissue is just one of the ways that muscle spasm impacts your health and well-being. Let's look at some others.

SPASM—A THREE-PRONGED PROBLEM

In order to realize the extent to which muscle influences your health, you must first understand the holistic nature of the body. Holistic is a word that has been so overused, it's easy to lose sight of its true meaning—that all parts of the body are dependent on each other, and that the body is constantly communicating with itself. Anything that affects one part of the body, affects the entire organism. Medicine, with its specialties, encourages the opposite view. It is practiced as if every organ were independent of the other, a very serious error.

Your body is such a sensitive instrument that it is influenced by and responds to everything it touches in any way. For instance, something as innocuous as a mild fluctuation in body temperature can produce many bodily reactions. Even radio waves, which are all around us all the time, have an effect, however subtle. So when any part of your body becomes irritated or dysfunctional, it will generally disturb other areas.

Because we are adaptable rather than stable organisms, our bodies are always reacting and shifting. We are influenced by everything that happens around us and all that happens inside of us. Since most of what is inside us is muscle, the excessive hardness and tension of hypertonic spasm is interpreted by the body as internal stress. Though you are not even aware it is there, spasm is affecting your health on three different fronts: circulatory, nerve, and orthopedic.

Circulatory Stress

Artery walls are very thick and will not ordinarily be compressed by spastic muscles. However, as we explained earlier in this chapter, constant stress on the arteries from lactic acid is a major factor in cholesterol plaquing and the blockage that may lead to heart attack.

Capillaries, venules, and veins *can* be constricted by spastic muscle. Just as a plant will wither if it's not watered, your body will suffer when its blood supply is hampered. Poor circulation can lead to a wide range of problems, from varicose veins to stroke.

Spasm can also make you look older. In fact, plastic surgeons do more face lifts on joggers and exercisers than on the rest of the population. When they searched for an explanation, they came up with the idea that bouncing causes gravity to pull a jogger's face down. But the real reason people who exercise heavily look prematurely old is that spasm is constricting their circulation.

In addition to making us look older, spasm can also cause us to die sooner. According to calculations based on the human gestation period, relative body size, and basal metabolism, we should be enjoying an average life expectancy of 150 years. One of the reasons we die before we should is that spasm impedes our circulation.

Nerve Stress

A spastic muscle is a hard muscle. For this reason, it can irritate any nerve it comes in contact with. When nerve irritation occurs as a result of a particular movement, the nervous system will automatically try to prevent further motion—whether or not you are conscious of pain. This is what causes stiffness, "catches," or a limited range of motion. An irritated nerve can also cause reluctance in the muscle, making it appear "weak" when it is actually overly contracted. When spastic, hardened muscle touches a nerve, the spasm may also bring on a *guarding reflex* that completely blocks movement. This is what happens when you bend over and can't straighten up again.

If spasm irritates nerves that are linked to internal organs such as the lungs or kidneys, it can cause problems in the function of those organs. Spasm can also have a powerful impact on your endocrine system and the function of your glands. This is why muscle spasm is a factor in many metabolic and autoimmune diseases.

Orthopedic Stress

The excess tension produced by spasm can cause changes in your body's structure. For instance, the tissue of a spastic muscle will become more fibrous, making the muscle harder, less flexible, and more susceptible to injury. In addition, spastic muscle will cause tendons to thicken. Over time, these tendons may eventually become calcified, or hardened by deposits of calcium. This can lead to spurs, which, contrary to popular belief, are accumulations in tendon, not on bone.

Spastic muscle can also compress your joint cartilage and spinal discs, making them thinner and more dense, and causing them to bulge. Doctors often mistake this protrusion for torn cartilage or a herniated disc. Spastic muscles can also pull your joints out of alignment.

Now that you know how muscle spasm develops, and the general ways in which it affects your health, let's get down to the details of just how spasm is involved in a host of illnesses and dysfunctions.

PART TWO
A Guide to Common Problems

You are about to learn exactly what may be wrong with you, what can cause your specific symptoms, and precisely which muscles are involved.

Though muscle is the most common cause of the conditions we will discuss, it may be advisable to see a doctor in order to rule out the possibility that something other than muscle is causing the problem, that a pain symptom, for instance, is not being caused by a tumor.

There are times, however, when your doctor's advice is based on insufficient training. I'm going to present some information which your doctor probably does not possess. This information is strong evidence against undergoing surgery for what many physicians erroneously label "torn rotator cuff," "torn medial meniscus knee cartilage," "carpal tunnel syndrome," and "herniated" or "slipped" disc. With some exceptions, it is also inadvisable to undergo hip replacement surgery. All of these conditions, and many others, can be corrected by releasing muscle spasm.

Doctors and chiropractors are at a loss in dealing with most of the symptoms we are about to discuss because they do not know what causes them. They have no understanding of muscle *dysfunction* because they have not learned how muscles *function*. What little they know of muscle involves only *structure*. Even medical books supposedly devoted to functional anatomy consider muscle as only part of the body's structure, and would more accurately be called "movement" anatomy books. They do not make the crucial, functional distinction between flat and round muscle, nor are they concerned with how muscles affect one another and the rest of the body.

Because medicine has taken so little interest in muscle, magnetic resonance imaging, or MRI, is useless in diagnosing many muscle-related conditions. It is a wonderful tool, but in order to interpret the data from an MRI, a computer program must be created. There are specific programs for many kinds of soft tissue, such as discs, ligaments, even the brain—but *no program has been developed to interpret MRI data on muscle.*

By the time you finish this part of the book, you'll know more than your doctor, chiropractor, or physical therapist about what causes a host of symptoms and common conditions. Even so, this is only an introduction to understanding muscles, a primer to allow the average person to grasp the essential findings drawn from twenty-five years of research and clinical experience. The information offered here has been extremely abbreviated in order to simplify its presentation.

In Chapter 4, we'll look at dysfunctions that are purely muscular, such as back, shoulder, neck, hip, and knee problems. In Chapter 5, we'll learn about the *suboccipital* muscles at the base of your skull, which are related to sinus problems, asthma, allergies, headaches, and more. They also play a key role in metabolic and autoimmune diseases. In Chapter 6, we'll see how muscle affects the health of many internal organs, including your heart, kidneys, and digestive and reproductive systems.

4

Muscles, Bones, and Joints

Whatever your particular complaint, it is important to understand that the source is rarely an isolated spasm in one part of your body alone. With a few exceptions, your symptom is part of an overall *pattern of spasticity*. People with lower back problems, for example, always have related tension in the shoulder, and often develop leg pain.

This pattern develops because round muscle goes bad in a kind of chain reaction. Since the body is holistic, and your muscles are interconnected, a spastic muscle can cause other muscles to spasm through interference with the blood supply, shared reflex nerves, or simply by contact. This chain of spastic muscle forms the same basic pattern in everyone. In fact, you'll find these same patterns even in animals. It is important to understand this, because when working with muscle, you must treat the whole pattern, not just the area in which the symptom has appeared.

Although every one of us has essentially the same spastic pattern, there will be certain variations within the pattern from individual to individual. Genetics, for instance, determine how close a muscle is to a nerve, or the diseases to which you are predisposed.

THE SKEWED-TORSO PATTERN— MISDIAGNOSIS: "SHORT-LEG SYNDROME"

All of us are lopsided. Go to the mirror, and you'll see what I mean. It may help if you cinch a belt around your waist. Look carefully, and you will observe that, to some degree, one side of the belt is higher than the other, giving the impression that one hip is higher. Now, look down at one leg of your pants or the hem of your dress. You'll notice that it hangs longer on the hip that appears lower, as if one leg were shorter than the other. The distortion is more pronounced in some people than in others, so even if you can't see it, trust me, you're lopsided.

If you were to lie down on a practitioner's table, the leg that appears shorter when you are standing would still look shorter. From this evidence, most chiropractors draw the conclusion that you do, indeed, have one short leg or that the leg has been shortened by what they'll call a "rotated" or uneven pelvis. A true short leg is extremely rare and is usually a congenital deformity. And the diagnosis "rotated" pelvis, like "slipped" disc, is incorrect. The real reason one leg *appears* shorter than the other is something else entirely. Let me show you proof.

Stand up and place a thumb on each hip where the bone protrudes in front. You'll see that your hip bones are perfectly level. If one of your legs were really shorter than the other, your hipbones (pelvis) would have to be uneven too. Why, then, is one leg shorter when you are lying down? Why is your belt lopsided? And why is the leg of your pants lower on one side?

What we have here is a skewed torso. Although the distortion *appears* to be vertical (i.e. a short leg), it's actually horizontal. What's *really* happening is that your torso is being pulled to one side by spastic muscles in the fleshy part of your hip, above your pelvis.

Now take a closer look at your hips. Notice that on the side where your waist *appears* higher, your hip protrudes more, and on the side where your waist *appears* lower, your hip looks somewhat flattened. This is why your belt and clothes are uneven—they slide down on the flat hip. Why, then, when you lie down, do your hipbones still *appear* uneven? The reason is that gravity is no longer anchoring you. Now, the same muscles that are pulling your torso to one side are pulling that hip toward your head.

Which muscles are involved, and why are they doing this? Let's see what is causing your torso to become skewed.

How You Became Lopsided

Whenever spastic muscles touch, they form a kind of mutual irritation society, not unlike some marriages. The *iliocostalis*, a long muscle that runs all the way from your shoulder down to a part of the pelvis called the *sacrum*, is highly susceptible to spasm. At the point where the iliocostalis attaches to the sacrum, it lies on top of the *multifidus to the third lumbar vertebra*. This muscle touches the *fourth lumbar nerve* very close to the root as shown in Figure 4.1. When the iliocostalis goads the multifidus into spasm, the lumbar nerve becomes trapped and extremely irritated. Some people experience this as a sharp pain in the lower back at the level of the *fifth lumbar vertebra*, but in most people the pain is numbed by endorphins.

Whether or not you feel pain, the nerve irritation is so intense, the body reacts by trying to pull the mulitfidus to the third lumbar away from the nerve. On the opposite side, in reaction, the *quadratus lumborum to the third lumbar vertebra* tenses and pulls the spine up and over. This lifts the multifidus to the third lumbar off the nerve.

In short, one muscle has to contract in order to pull

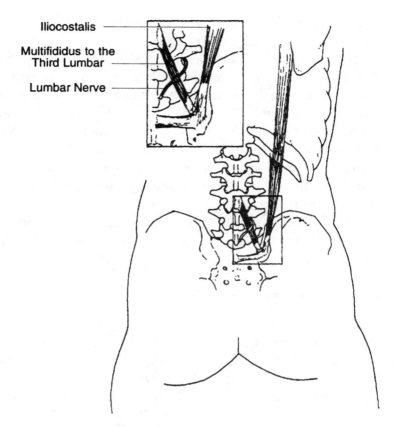

Iliocostalis

Multifididus to the
Third Lumbar

Lumbar Nerve

Figure 4.1. The Beginning of the Skewed Torso. The iliocostalis carries irritation from the shoulder down to the multifidus to the third lumbar. The spastic multifidus to the third lumbar, in turn, pinches the fourth lumbar nerve causing pain.

another muscle away from a nerve. This is called a *guarding reflex*, shown in Figure 4.2. In order to avoid pain, the pulling muscle cannot let up its guard; it must remain contracted. Eventually, lactic acid builds up, and the muscle becomes chronically spastic. This permanent spasm keeps your body pulled to one side, skewing your torso and creating the lopsided look. Both your legs are the same length, but the side doing the pulling *appears* lower. Frequently, this guarding reflex recruits the *psoas* muscle, which runs

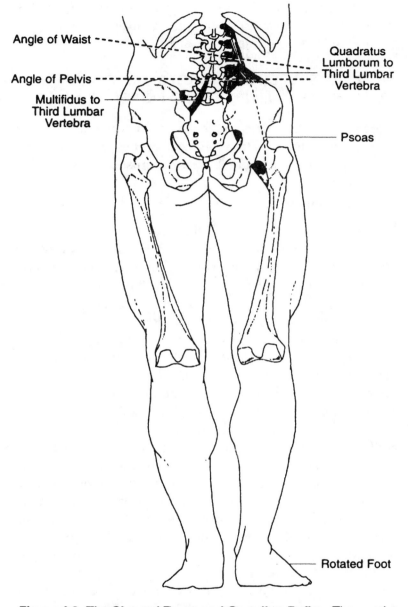

Angle of Waist

Angle of Pelvis

Multifidus to
Third Lumbar
Vertebra

Quadratus
Lumborum to
Third Lumbar
Vertebra

Psoas

Rotated Foot

Figure 4.2. The Skewed Torso and Guarding Reflex. The quadratus lumborum to the third lumbar pulls the spine over to lift the multifidus to the third lumbar off the lumbar nerve. As a result, the waist becomes uneven, but the pelvis remains level.

from the front upper thigh to the spine. You can see that the psoas has become spastic when the foot on the pulling or "short leg" side is rotated outward.

MUSCULOSKELETAL DISORDERS THAT ARE PART OF THE SKEWED-TORSO PATTERN

The following disorders are, for the most part, related to the basic skewed-torso pattern. To correct these problems, the entire pattern, not just one local area, must be massaged.

Shoulder Tension

You may be aware of the fact that one of your shoulders is chronically more tense than the other. This is true for everyone. The chronically spastic shoulder is always on the same side as the spastic multifidus to the third lumbar vertebra—the side with the protruding hip, the side your body is being pulled away from. Because the shoulder is highly vulnerable to spasm, the skewed-torso pattern often begins here.

Shoulder muscles are most often irritated by a muscle virus that attacks the upper portion of the iliocostalis. There is a specific virus for each shoulder, so you will usually experience an attack on only one side. However, you won't find any mention of shoulder viruses in medical textbooks. Their existence is an inescapable conclusion drawn from years of observing a distinct type of local shoulder pain that behaves exactly like any other virus.

There are two types of shoulder viruses: *indigenous* and *contagious*. Indigenous viruses are in our bodies all the time, and they will attack when we are run down or otherwise physically vulnerable. That's why, when some people lose a night's sleep, or undergo other kinds of stress that affect the immune system, they experience a sudden sharp pain in the shoulder, upper back, or neck. The chronically tense shoulder is more susceptible to indigenous viruses. Contagious shoulder viruses, on the other hand, travel from person to person just like flu bugs. And they are more virulent than indigenous viruses. What else but a virus could cause my office to suddenly fill up with people, all complaining of pain in the same shoulder?

The *trapezius* muscles, which run from the neck to the shoulders to the mid-back, generally take the blame for shoulder tension. But, except for one small, round section, the trapezius muscles are flat and cannot become spastic. A massage that tries to relieve shoulder tension by plunging into the trapezius, pinching, squeezing, and poking, may bring on endorphins for temporary relief. However, this type of treatment will probably create spasm in the muscles below the trapezius—the *serratus anterior*, and the muscles it abuts, the iliocostalis, and the *scalenes*, seen in Figure 4.3.

Eventually, shoulder viruses create a chronically spastic iliocastalis, spreading spasm to many other muscles. This is how many of the problems connected with the skewed-torso pattern begin.

The Upper Back: "Catches" and "Pins"

A shoulder virus can cause a "catch"—pain that interrupts motion—in the upper back. This is how it happens.

The last digitation of the serratus anterior puts stress on the eighth rib. Because of this, the *eighth intercostal muscle* bulges out beyond the other intercostals. (Intercostals are muscles between ribs.) The iliocostalis crosses over and can irritate the bulging eighth intercostal, causing you to feel a "catch" just inside the lower part of the shoulder blade, as shown in Figure 4.4.

Chiropractors will often diagnose this symptom as a slight structural misalignment, an incomplete dislocation, a "rotated rib," or a rib that's "out." In the course of trying to correct what they believe is a rib problem, chiropractors may further irritate the eighth intercostal muscle.

When other muscles in the back are spastic and touch a

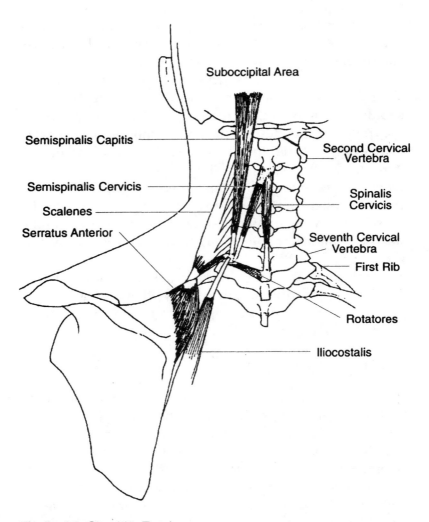

Figure 4.3. Shoulder Tension.

nerve, you may feel like there's a "pin" running right
through your fifth vertebra, clear through to your *sternum*,
or breastbone. Sometimes you see people thrusting their
shoulders back and sticking out their chests trying to get
rid of this pain. Here's what causes it.

The iliocostalis passes under and irritates a round portion of the trapezius muscle, which runs from the inside edge of the middle of the shoulder blade to the back of the fifth thoracic vertebra (T5), as shown in Figure 4.4. This irritation causes a pulling on the attachment at T5, putting stress on the *sixth intercostal muscle*. The sixth intercostal is then further irritated where it contacts the iliocostalis just before the intercostal runs under the shoulder blade.

The reason the "pin" pain seems to go through the body is that the sixth intercostal runs all the way around from the back to the front of the body—but is felt at the center of the muscle arc, providing something akin to stereo reception. This tendency of "nerve summation" is how the body allows you to feel things beyond itself, just as it does when you're writing and can feel the tip of the pen.

A Crick in the Neck

The center of a shoulder virus attack—the iliocostalis where it attaches to the side of the *seventh cervical vertebra*—is most often numbed by endorphins. But the iliocostalis attachment can, by contact, irritate the *semispinalis cervicis* and the *rotatores*. Spasm in the semispinalis cervicis and the rotatores may give you a crick in the neck near the back of the seventh cervical vertebra. As shown in Figure 4.3, the spastic rotatores carries tension directly to the back of the seventh vertebra while the semispinalis cervicis takes it to the back of the *second cervical vertebra* and then down to the seventh vertebra via the *spinalis cervicis*. Most people blame this type of neck pain on the way they've slept, but it is actually brought on by a shoulder virus.

A crick in the neck is often accompanied by a tension headache because the spastic iliocostalis contacts and irritates the *semispinalis capitis*, which runs up to the suboccipital area at the base of the skull.

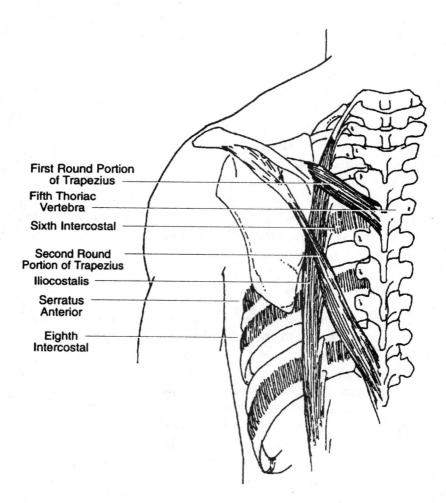

First Round Portion
   of Trapezius

Fifth Thoriac
   Vertebra

Sixth Intercostal

Second Round
Portion of Trapezius

Iliocostalis

Serratus
Anterior

Eighth
Intercostal

Figure 4.4. "Catches" and "Pins."

Stiff Neck

The crick in the neck mentioned above can irritate the lower attachment of the *splenius capitis* muscle, shown in Figure 4.5.

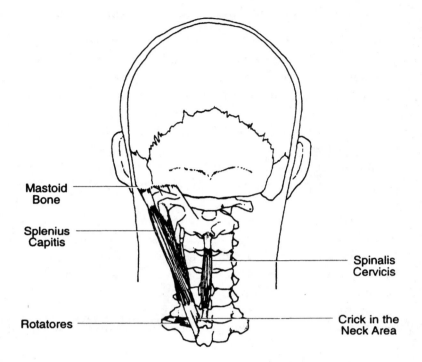

Mastoid Bone

Splenius Capitis

Rotatores

Spinalis Cervicis

Crick in the Neck Area

Figure 4.5. Stiff Neck. The crick in the neck can become a stiff neck at the attachment of the splenius capitis.

A spastic splenius capitis creates the "new" stiff neck, the kind that prevents you from turning your head to one side. I say "new" because thirty or forty years ago, when you had a stiff neck, you would be frozen looking to one side. This was caused by a virus called the *torticollus* that affected the *sternocleidomastoid* (seen in Figure 4.6), the muscle that pulls the *mastoid bone* toward the sternum. That virus has now become quite rare. But I once had a client who was born with chronic spasm in the sternocleidomastoid. When he was still an infant, the doctors cut partially through the muscle to weaken it so that he would be able to turn his head. Instead of performing surgery on a newborn baby, the doctors could have released the muscle with massage.

Dizziness, Facial Pain, Ringing in the Ears, and Tics

A spastic splenius capitis muscle can also cause dizziness, facial pain, ringing in the ears, and tics. The splenius capitis attaches to the tip of the mastoid bone next to and in contact with the *digastric* muscle, as shown in Figure 4.6. The contact of the splenius capitis with the digastric can make the digastric spastic. The function of the digastric is to help elevate your voice box when you speak. It sits right on top of a group of nerves which includes the *trigeminal nerve*, the *stato-acoustic nerve*, and the *facial nerve*.

Here's what can happen when these nerves become irritated. The acoustic nerve can cause ringing in the ears (not to be mistaken for *tinnitus*, a buzzing or ringing caused by pressure in the inner ear). The stato portion of the stato-acoustic nerve can produce dizziness or nausea. The trigeminal nerve can cause facial pain. And irritation in the facial nerve can bring about uncontrolled muscular contractions, or tics.

Throat and Thyroid Problems

The sternocleidomastoid, splenius capitis, and digastric all share an attachment. This creates what you might call a *ménage à trois* of spastic muscles, seen in Figure 4.6. The sternocleidomastoid presses against the throat muscles, and when it is spastic it can produce a sore or tickling throat which is easily irritated when you speak.

A spastic sternocleidomastoid muscle may also cause circulation problems around the thyroid gland. While the pituitary gland is responsible for controlling thyroid function and the suboccipital muscles at the base of the skull (which we will discuss in the next chapter) have the most powerful effect on the pituitary, working the sternocleidomastoid muscle can still help some thyroid problems.

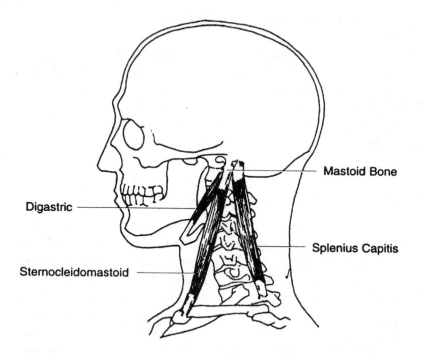

Mastoid Bone

Digastric

Splenius Capitis

Sternocleidomastoid

Figure 4.6. Ménage à Trois. An irritated digastric muscle can cause dizziness, facial pain, ringing in the ears, and tics. A muscular ménage à trois is created by a shared attachment of the digastric, sternocleidomastoid, and splenius capitis. The shared attachment causes irritation in the sternocleidomastoid, leading to head, throat, and thyroid problems.

Bell's Palsy

Bell's palsy is caused by a virus that attacks the digastric muscle (seen in Figure 4.6), which then pushes into the facial nerve. This results in a loss of control of the muscles on one side of the face, which go completely limp, creating a lopsided look.

The conventional treatment for Bell's palsy is to leave it alone and let it go away on its own. This doesn't always work. I have had clients come to me saying, "The doctor told me I would be fine in six weeks. That was three years ago, and my face is still distorted." I've also seen people who have experienced the residual effects of Bell's palsy for twenty years!

Bell's palsy can be completely reversed by massaging the digastric and other muscles in the pattern, as well as the involved facial muscles. Many people recover in six weeks, but even that is an unnecessarily long recovery period. With treatment, all Bell's palsy symptoms can be gone in a week.

Lower-Back Pain

The muscles at the core of the skewed-torso pattern—the iliocostalis, the multifidus to the third lumbar, and the quadratus lumborum to the third lumbar on the opposite side—are the source of most lower-back pain. By the time your muscles have begun pulling to one side, endorphins are already numbing you, so only a small percentage of people actually feel the sharp pain from the fourth lumbar nerve on the side being pulled. A greater number of people experience lower-back pain on the pulling side, but don't realize that there is also chronic spasm on the opposite side—the side being pulled. In order to release spasm in the lower back, it is necessary to work the iliocostalis not just at the sacrum, but at the shoulder as well.

Other muscles also contribute to lower-back pain. The quadratus lumborum to the third lumbar attaches to the top rear of the pelvic bone, right next to the attachment of a round portion of the *gluteus medius*, as shown in Figure 4.7. Both of these muscles irritate each other. The gluteus medius, a combination of flat and round muscle, runs from the *ilium*, which forms each side of the pelvis, to the outer portion of the upper thigh, where it attaches to the *femur*, or thigh bone. The attachment line of the gluteus medius carries irritation forward to the *sartorius* and *tensor fascia lata* muscles of the leg.

(Incidentally, there are two other gluteus muscles: the

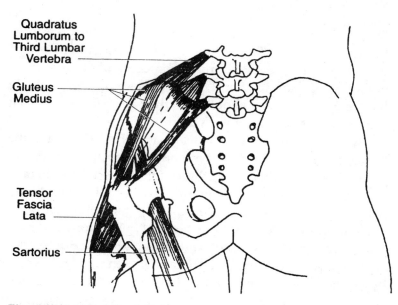

Figure 4.7. Lower Back Pain.

gluteus minimus and the gluteus maximus. The gluteus minimus is partly round and susceptible to spasm. But the gluteus maximus is primarily flat—luckily, since we sit on it. If the gluteus maximus were susceptible to spasm, we'd be in a lot of trouble.)

Getting Stuck in a Bent-Over Position

Have you ever bent over too quickly, then been unable to stand up straight again? Here's why. A spastic iliocostalis is not capable of suddenly stretching out. If you move too fast, it will press into the multifidus to the third lumbar, forcing it against the fourth lumbar nerve. The pressure is so sudden, there's no time to build up endorphins against it. First you feel a sharp stabbing pain, then the muscles "freeze" to avoid any more pain.

Spinal Discs

One of the most common—and dangerous—mistakes doctors make is diagnosing a "herniated," degenerated, or torn vertebral disc. There is so much confusion about discs that before we go any further, I'd like to clear up some widely held misconceptions about how they function, and what can and can't go wrong with them.

According to *Gray's Anatomy*, vertebral discs are the "chief bonds" holding the vertebrae together. Discs *do not* act as shock absorbers or cushions for the vertebrae. In fact, they move with them. They are also very durable. Many people (and doctors, too, I'm afraid) think that a disc is something like a jelly donut—a sac of gel surrounded by a thin membrane, as seen in Figure 4.8 (A). But *Gray's Anatomy* tells us that after the age of ten, the gel center becomes fibrocartilage—an extremely durable material, shown in Figure 4.8 (B). In fact, in engineering terms, fibrocartilage is as sturdy as prestressed concrete—a material used to build bridges! Moreover, the fibrocartilage in discs is surrounded by hyaline cartilage, a substance as friction-free as Teflon that prevents the vertebrae and discs from touching—and makes wear and tear on the disc virtually impossible.

If it's almost impossible for a vertebral disc to degenerate, why do doctors keep looking at x-rays and diagnosing herniated discs? Because they don't know what they are looking at. What they see on an x-ray is a diminished space between the vertebrae. Then, because they have no other explanation, they mistakenly conclude that the disc is degenerated. But if they took the action of muscles into consideration, they would see that spastic muscles are exerting pressure on the vertebrae, compressing the discs. For instance, Figure 4.9 shows how spastic psoas muscles can compress the lumbar discs, flattening the normal back curve. Similarly, the scalenes can compress the cervical discs, flattening the normal neck curve.

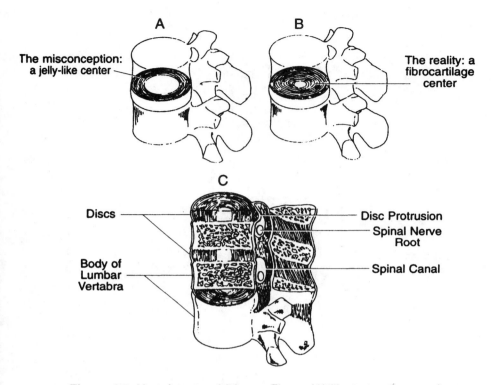

Figure 4.8. Vertebrae and Discs. Figure (A) illustrates the popular misconception that a disc has a jelly-like center which acts as a cushion between vertebrae. Figure (B) shows the reality—a strong fibrocartilage center. Figure (C) shows the body of the lumbar verte-bra and vertebral discs in cross-section. Even if a squashed disc were to extrude well into the spinal canal it would occupy less than half of the exit—so it is unlikely to exert pressure on the nerve root.

One result of disc compression is that a portion of the disc begins to protrude. Again, doctors do not understand what they are seeing. They often diagnose the protrusion as a herniation, or tear, and recommend disc surgery. But disc surgery is not only completely unnecessary, it is also extremely dangerous. Arteries and nerves can be negative-ly affected, even severed. If surgery is performed in the thoracic region (the middle to upper back), there is also considerable risk of paralysis. This is even more horrifying when you realize that, according to the study cited in

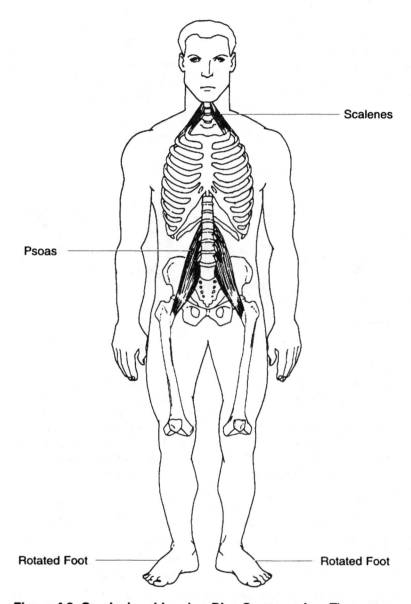

Figure 4.9. Cervical and Lumbar Disc Compression. The powerful psoas muscles can apply compressive force to the lumbar discs, flattening the back and rotating the legs and feet outward. Similarly, the scalenes can apply compressive force to the cervical discs, flattening the neck curve.

Chapter 2, a true herniated disc is so rare as to be virtually nonexistent.

Arm and Hand Problems— Misdiagnosis: "Herniated Cervical Disc"

When patients present symptoms of numbness, tingling, pain, and weakness in the arms and hands, doctors often make a diagnosis of "herniated cervical disc" or "degenerative disc disease," then run for the scalpel. But a cervical disc that *appears* to be protruding in an x-ray is almost always a disc that has been compressed because of spasm in the scalene muscles, as seen in Figure 4.9. Sometimes, when a doctor diagnoses a cervical disc problem, an MRI will show that there's nothing wrong with the disc. So the doctor may come up with another diagnosis—thoracic outlet—and remove the first rib. Thoracic outlet is based on the mistaken idea that the rib is in the way of the opening between it and the second rib, pinching the nerve slightly below the disc area. It's true that the nerve is being irritated—but not by the rib.

Numbness, tingling, pain, or weakness in the arms and hands may have several different causes. Sometimes a spastic iliocostalis makes contact with the serratus anterior near the serratus attachment to the upper shoulder blade. The serratus anterior, in turn, makes contact with the *scalenus posterior*, which surrounds the *brachial plexus*, a complex of nerves that travels into the shoulder, arm, and hand, as shown in Figure 4.10. A spastic scalenus posterior muscle can cause tingling, numbness, or pain in the arm by irritating nerve trunks.

Frequently, arm and hand pain is caused by the brachialis or the *triceps* muscle of the upper arm pressing into the nerve further down, as seen in Figure 4.10. Tingling, numbness, or pain in the thumb side of the hand most often is caused by irritation of the *median nerve* by the brachialis muscle. The same symptoms in the pinky and ring fingers usually occur when the medial, or middle, head of the tri-

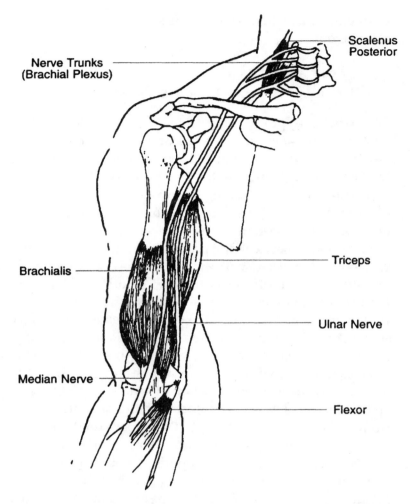

Figure 4.10. Pain in the Arm and Hand. Spastic scalenus posterior, brachialis, triceps, and forearm flexor muscles conspire to irritate nerves, causing pain in the arms and hands.

ceps irritates the *ulnar nerve.* Frequently, the source of hand and arm discomfort is the *extensor, flexor,* or *supinator* muscles in forearm or hand. For example, "funny bone" pain occurs when the flexor muscle irritates the ulnar nerve. I'll discuss these muscles further when we look at "tennis elbow."

Buttock and Leg Pain—
Misdiagnosis: " Herniated Lumbar Disc"

When patients complain of pain in the buttocks or legs, doctors sometimes take an MRI, see a protruding disc, and jump to the erroneous conclusion that the disc is herniated. Then they want to operate.

Here's what's *really* causing the problem. When the quadratus lumborum to the third lumbar pulls your torso to one side, it may also enlist the help of the psoas muscle, which runs from the first lumbar vertebra, just below the rib, down to the top of the thigh bone. When the psoas contracts, it exerts a downward force which can cause the discs to compress. This pressure makes the disc protrude—not herniate—and it will protrude farther on the pulling side of the torso. The disc is *not* degenerated. In fact, it is made more dense by compression.

It is highly unlikely, however, that this protrusion causes the pain. The spinal cord proper ends at the bottom of the rib cage, and the lumbar spine openings are several times larger than the exiting nerve roots, so a protruding disc will rarely disturb nerve root function, as seen in Figure 4.8(C). The pain usually comes from the nerve trunk, which can be irritated by any number of spastic muscles in the lower body.

Another problem accompanying disc compression is a flattened back. The psoas attaches to the front of the spine, then comes forward to the leg bone. When it tightens, it acts just like a bowstring, pulling your pelvis forward, making your buttocks turn under, as shown in Figure 4.11. A contracted psoas will not only flatten your back, causing strain at the lumbosacral joint (at the base of the spine), it will also make your foot turn outward.

Iliotibial-Tract Pain—Misdiagnosis: Sciatica

Although sciatic pain is one of the most common, catch-all

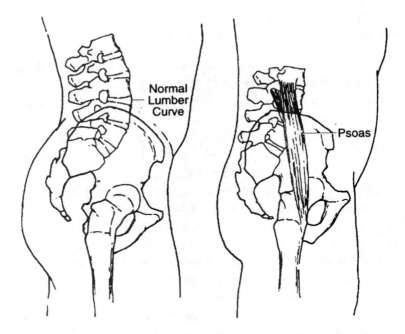

Figure 4.11. Buttock and Leg Pain. Spastic psoas muscles compress lumbar discs, pulling the pelvis forward and making the buttocks turn under. This can cause pain in the buttocks or legs.

diagnoses for pain running from the buttocks down the leg, true sciatic pain is rare. When pain does come from the sciatic nerve, it starts near the middle of the buttocks—more than an inch inward from where people diagnosed with sciatica usually feel pain. Chiropractors and doctors will often associate sciatic pain with a muscle called the *piriformis* (located at the midpoint of each buttock). This is because the sciatic nerve passes through this muscle in some people, but it is fairly rare.

In most people, the sciatic nerve passes through a notch between the piriformis and the *gemellus superior* muscles (just below the periformis) then immediately toward the foot, over the attachment of the gemellus superior, as seen in Figure 4.12. The gemellus is a flat muscle, but it does become spastic at its attachment. However, this spasm

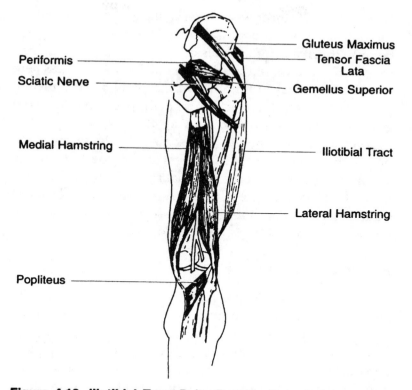

Periformis

Sciatic Nerve

Medial Hamstring

Popliteus

Gluteus Maximus

Tensor Fascia Lata

Gemellus Superior

Iliotibial Tract

Lateral Hamstring

Figure 4.12. Iliotibial Tract Pain. Because the sciatic nerve lies close to the iliotibial tract, iliotibial tract pain is often misdiagnosed as sciatica.

must be quite intense before it comes into contact with the nerve. When it does, it can cause true sciatic pain, but the condition is not common and is always accompanied by iliotibial tract pain.

The *iliotibial tract* begins a few inches below the top of the pelvis, near the *sacroiliac joint*, at the upper border of the gluteus maximus, which abuts the iliocostalis over the sacroiliac joint. The tract then runs out and down the side of the hip and leg. Sometimes this tract is numb; at other times it is extremely tender and painful when probed.

The iliotibial tract is made up of three parts: anterior, medial, and posterior. The posterior portion of the iliotibial

tract, formed by the lower border of the gluteus maximus, is
the one most easily confused with the site of sciatic pain
because it runs along the outside back of the thigh, an inch
or so to the outside of the sciatic nerve. Pain or stiffness here
can also be mistaken for a hamstring problem. The medial
portion of the iliotibial tract begins at the upper border of the
gluteus maximus. Almost midway to the knee, the tract
overlies a series of nerves that sometimes cause pain, but
more commonly produce numbness on the side of the thigh.
The anterior portion of the iliotibial tract is formed from the
tensor fascia lata muscle which, as discussed before, can contribute to a feeling of stiffness in the hip. Below the knee, the
sciatic and iliotibial tracts merge into one.

Hip Problems

Limited motion of the hip and dysfunction of the hip joint
are often treated with surgery, but the cause of these problems is usually spastic muscles.

The quadratus lumborum to the third lumbar vertebra,
one of the primary muscles involved in the skewed-torso
pattern, irritates the gluteus medius near the forward edge
of the pelvis. This, in turn, creates spasticity in the tensor
fascia lata (in the hip) and the sartorius (in the thigh). The
sartorius, the longest muscle in your body, runs down
along the inside of the *quadriceps*, or thigh muscles, and
attaches to the inside of the knee, as shown in Figure 4.13.
If your sartorius muscle has become irritated, you will
appear to bend forward when standing, as if you were
leaning into the wind. Because the sartorius crosses over
the hip joint itself, chronic spasm in this muscle may eventually reduce the range of motion of the hip. The sartorius
also passes over and can irritate the *adductor longus* (in the
lower groin), limiting the side extension of the leg, either
with or without pain.

Spasticity in the tensor fascia lata muscle, which works
with the sartorius to lift the leg, also plays a role in hip-joint

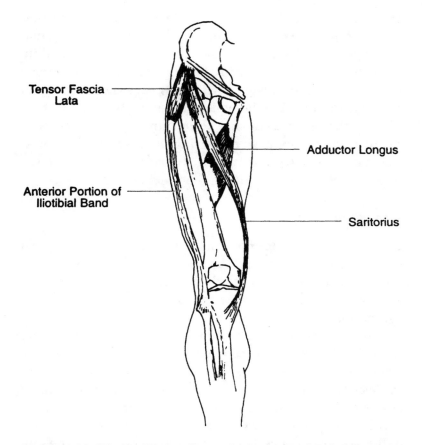

Figure 4.13. Hip Problems. Spasm in the tensor fascia lata, sartorius, and adductor longus muscles can limit hip movement and cause you to bend forward.

problems. When movement in the hip joint becomes impaired, doctors frequently prescribe hip replacement surgery, although these symptoms usually have nothing to do with the hip joint itself. As chronic spastic tension worsens, the muscles around the hip joint—not the joint itself—become calcified. This can be seen quite clearly in x-rays. With the exception of people with congenital hip problems, there is much less need for hip replacement surgery than is presently being done. I have worked on many people who were told by doctors that they needed hip surgery, yet their x-rays showed good, smooth, round bones, which still had cartilage between them. The cartilage was very thin, because it had been compressed by tension from spastic muscles. But compressed cartilage is very dense, so it can still perform its job quite well. It takes many years of spasticity in the sartorius muscle before you lose your ability to move at the hip joint, so correcting the problem with massage takes some time. However, the range of motion usually increases noticeably after a few treatments.

Knee Pain

One of the most common diagnoses of knee pain is torn *medial meniscus* cartilage, and the suggested remedy is often surgery. But of all the clients I have treated who have been so diagnosed, not one needed surgery to eliminate the symptoms.

We all have tiny tears in the medial meniscus cartilage, located at the center of the knee, but those tears are not the problem. In fact, many people diagnosed with torn medial meniscus cartilage do not even experience pain or swelling at the level of the knee joint. The most common site of pain, because it is part of the skewed-torso pattern, is on the inside of the knee just below the joint at the attachment of the sartorius muscle and tendon, as shown in Figure 4.14. This is also the attachment of the medial hamstring (at the back of the thigh), which wraps around the knee and attaches in front, below the knee joint. This shared attachment of the medial hamstring and the sartorius can cause pain in the area of the medial meniscus cartilage. Pain can also occur at the upper attachment of the sartorius where it abuts the iliotibial tract. Sometimes the attachment of the iliotibial tract also causes pain on the outside of the knee just below the joint.

Other knee problems are independent of the skewed-torso pattern. These involve three of the four thigh muscles of the quadriceps group. The *rectus* is flat and therefore not

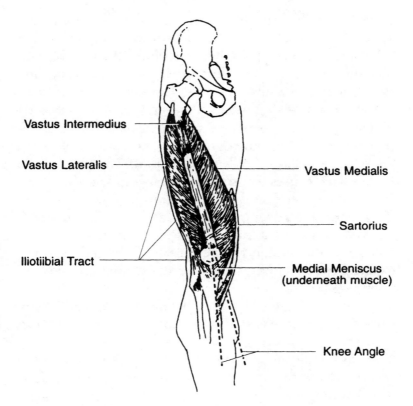

Figure 4.14. Knee Pain. The sartorius, vastus lateralis, vastus medialis, vastus intermedius, and the attachment of the iliotibial tract conspire to produce pain in the knee, some of which is part of the skewed-torso pattern and some of which is independent of it.

part of the problem, but the *vastus medialis, vastus intermedius,* and *vastus lateralis* are all round and very prone to spasm.

Pain in the area of the medial meniscus cartilage can also be caused by a spastic vastus medialis muscle and tendon, shown in Figure 4.14, which can trap nerves at the knee joint. Because the thigh bone angles inward from hip to knee, forming an angle at the knee, the vastus medialis has to wrap around the angle to attach. This can cause a great deal of tension, which may irritate the nerves beneath the muscle.

Pain on the outside of the knee may be caused by a
spastic vastus lateralis. This occurs less frequently than
other types of knee pain, because unlike the vastus medialis, the vastus lateralis, seen in Figure 4.14, attaches in a
direct line. This allows the lateralis to endure more stress
without compressing nerves. So even when the vastus lateralis experiences a great deal of spasticity, you are less
likely to feel it. If, when you flex your knee, you hear a
"pop" or a "click," you've got a spastic vastus lateralis.
Here's what causes that sound. Watch your kneecap as you
flex your leg, and you'll see that, because of the angle of the
thigh bone, the kneecap moves sideways to the outside of
the knee. As it does this, it rides over the vastus lateralis
tendon. If the tendon has become hard, the kneecap will
experience resistance going over the tendon and create a
"popping" sound.

Pain immediately above or below the knee cap may be
caused by a spastic vastus intermedius, as shown in Figure
4.14.

Pain behind your knee stems from a spastic *popliteus*
muscle. The function of this muscle is to keep your knee
from bending backward. I once had a client, a famous skier,
whose popliteus muscles were so spastic, she would amaze
people at parties by popping her knees out behind her.
After I relaxed those muscles, she lost this startling ability.

These knee problems can be corrected by massaging
the individual muscles that are spastic.

However, unnecessary knee surgery is still widely practiced. Arthroscopic surgery, which involves only tiny inci-
sions, is frequently used now and results in less scarring
and restriction of the range of motion than more invasive
surgery. Yet despite these improved techniques, I still treat
many people who did not achieve the desired results after
surgery, and continued to suffer from pain, loss of feeling,
buckling or locked knees, or other symptoms for which they
had sought help. This is because surgery does not address
the real problem, which is in the muscles and tendons.

Doctors are simply doing what they have been trained to do. These harmful practices are bound to continue until medical schools begin to teach doctors what they need to know about muscle and the problems caused by its dysfunction.

The Calf and Foot

Many conditions involving the foot and calf involve spastic muscle. Surgery and drugs are common solutions, but they do not address the root of the problems—spastic muscle. The spastic muscles that cause the following disorders can be successfully treated with massage.

Cramps, Shin Splints, Varicose Veins, and Blood Clots

Below the knee, the iliotibial tract shares an attachment with the *peroneus* muscle and can irritate it. The peroneus muscle, which sits on the *peroneal nerve*, travels down the leg, then around the side of the foot, and finally attaches across the base of the toe muscles. This is the usual source of leg and toe cramps.

The peroneal nerve also feeds the *tibialis anterior* muscle (running parallel to the shin bone), which, when spastic, can give you shin splints (pain in the lower leg next to the shin bone caused by cramping after exercise). It can also cause pain in the main arch of the foot. A spastic *adductor hallucis transversum* (running across the bottom of the foot near the toes) may cause pain, burning, and a tired feeling in the metatarsal arch (running across the bottom of the foot near the toes).

The *soleus* muscle (shown in Figure 4.15) lies under the flat *gastrocnemius* in the calf. This is the only place in the body where a vein itself is actually routed through a muscle. As a result, the soleus muscle is a powerful venous pump, responsible for pumping the blood in the veins of the calf back up to the heart.

When spasm blocks this action, constricted venous drainage can produce leg cramps. If the deep veins become too constricted, they must be bypassed. This overloads the superficial veins, causing varicose veins—abnormally swollen and twisted blood vessels.

Spasticity in the soleus muscle, shown in Figure 4.15, can also cause blood clotting in the calf. These clots are not usually a problem, unless they travel above the knee joint. When they do, they can cause stroke, heart attack, or pulmonary embolism (a blood clot of a lung artery).

Bunions

The *extensor hallucis brevis* muscle, which runs from the top of the outside part of the foot to the big toe, can pull on the big toe and cause pain on top of the foot. It can also contribute to the formation of a bunion, an inflammation and swelling of

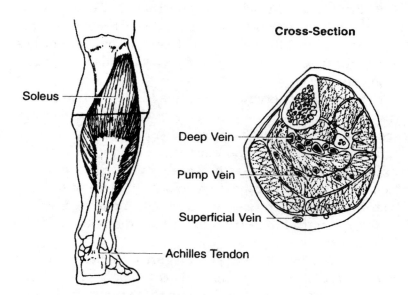

Figure 4.15. Leg Cramps and Varicose Veins. A spastic soleus constricts venous drainage in deep veins of the leg. This produces leg cramps and varicosis in overloaded superficial leg veins.

the big toe joint, although spastic failure of the *abductor hallucis* is usually the primary cause of this condition.

Fungal Toenails and Gangrene

It is commonly assumed that fungal toenails are an inevitable complication of the poor circulation common in patients with advanced diabetes. One reason for poor circulation in diabetics is an overproduction of histamine, which causes the membrane around the arteries to harden and thicken, choking off the blood supply. As you'll see in Chapter 5, histamine production can be controlled by releasing spasm in the suboccipital muscles at the base of the skull.

The other cause of poor circulation leading to fungal toenails is spasm in the muscles of the calf. When the condition becomes extreme, gangrene, the decay of tissue due to lack of blood supply, may develop. With massage, I have been able to bring gangrenous legs back to normal when doctors had called for immediate amputation.

Ankle Problems

The *tibialis anterior* muscle in the front of the calf and the *peroneus longus* muscle, on the outside of the calf, are the muscles that stabilize the ankle. If you have weak or wobbly ankles, it is probably because these muscles have too much tone, not too little.

When people strain and sprain their ankles, they are often told to ice them down. This is usually a bad idea because ice is a thermal shock to the muscles and will cause them to become spastic. Moreover, ice will stop the inflammation process, which is actually the healing process. When you first sprain an ankle, you should not automatically apply ice. Use ice only if the ankle becomes so swollen that the skin turns shiny. This indicates that the swelling and pressure have begun to block circulation and hamper healing. As soon as the skin loses its shine, stop icing it and let the healing run its course. After the ankle has healed on its own for a few days, the residual spasticity can be released with massage.

MUSCULOSKELETAL DISORDERS THAT ARE INDEPENDENT OF THE SKEWED-TORSO PATTERN

The following conditions involve standard muscle patterns that are not primarily related to the skewed-torso pattern. To correct these conditions, the individual patterns should be massaged. In addition, working with the skewed-torso pattern can also aid healing by reducing overall irritation to the nervous system.

Misdiagnosis: "Bone" Spurs and Osteoarthritis

Rheumatoid arthritis is a disease of the autoimmune system which involves true degeneration of the joints, and will be discussed in the next section.

It is often confused with a much more common condition that doctors call *osteoarthritis*. This is an ill-chosen name, because *osteo* means related to bone, but the symptoms have nothing to do with bone; and arthritis means joint inflammation, but there are no inflamed joints. The cause of osteoarthritis, or bone spurs, is calcified tendons. That's what makes fingers crooked and knobby.

Not long ago, doctors looking at motion picture x-rays of "bone spurs" saw them waving like flags in the breeze, following the motion of the tendon. Since tendons don't show up on x-rays, and bones don't move this way, the doctors were mystified by what they saw. They just sort of scratched their heads and thought it was odd. It never occurred to them that what they were watching wasn't bone at all, but calcified tendon. They were so intent upon maintaining their beliefs, that they clung to them even when staring at clear evidence that they were wrong.

When you release the spastic muscles involved in producing "bone" spurs and osteoarthritis, the reaction that caused the calcium to deposit will reverse.

Misdiagnosis: "Carpal Tunnel Syndrome"

The symptoms of the condition referred to as "carpal tunnel syndrome" are weakness, pain, or numbness in the wrist and thumb side of the hand. The condition can become quite acute, almost crippling.

Surgeons will tell you that you are in pain because the carpal "ligament," at the base of the palm, is impinging on the median nerve. But what surgeons call the carpal "ligament" is actually the carpal retinaculum—and it has absolutely nothing to do with the problem.

What *really* happens is that a bulging, spastic tendon of the thumb muscle, the *flexor pollicus longus* shown in Figure 4.16, presses into the nerve, trapping it against the finger tendons.

"Carpal tunnel syndrome" clears up quickly after a few massage treatments have released the spasm.

Misdiagnosis: "Temporomandibular Joint Syndrome" or TMJ

Doctors, chiropractors, dentists, dental surgeons, and orthodontists refer to most jaw pain as "temporomandibular joint syndrome" (TMJ). In doing so, they mistakenly attribute pain in the jaw to unusual stress being exerted on the *temporomandibular joint*. This is consistent with a structural rather than a functional approach. They treat the problem with surgery, bite plates, or "cracking" of the jaw to try to correct the assumed structural problem. Occasionally this results in the numbing of pain by endorphins, but no real improvement.

Most jaw pain is not caused by a joint, but by a muscle—the *temporalis*. The tempoalis muscle attaches to the *coronoid process* of the jaw just under the arch of the cheek,

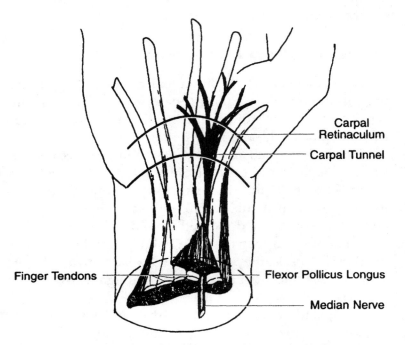

**Carpal
Retinaculum**

Carpal Tunnel

Finger Tendons

Flexor Pollicus Longus

Median Nerve

Figure 4.16. "Carpal Tunnel Syndrome." The flexor pollicus longus presses against the median nerve producing pain in the wrist and hand in what is often misdiagnosed "carpal tunnel syndrome."

as seen in Figure 4.17. Pain is felt at the coronoid process because the attachment of the temporalis to the jawbone becomes spastic and rubs against the inside of the cheekbone. The spastic temporalis can also cause the jaw to sit to the side or back of its proper bite.

Spasm in the temporalis can be released with massage.

Misdiagnosis: "Torn Rotator Cuff"

In the old days doctors called it bursitis and gave you a shot of cortisone. Today they will tell you it's a torn rotator cuff. Both diagnoses are wrong. You just have spastic muscles. Every diagnosed case of "torn rotator cuff" I have seen

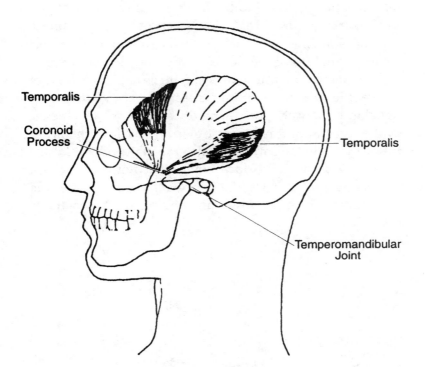

Figure 4.17. "TMJ." Jaw pain at the coronoid process caused by a spastic temporalis muscle is often misdiagnosed "temporomandibular joint syndrome."

responded to massage treatment without cortisone or surgery.

The symptoms are pain in the front of the shoulder, especially when you raise your arm to the side and rotate your wrist clockwise. The symptoms also include difficulty reaching far forward or behind. If the condition is especially bad, you may not be able to reach around into your back pocket.

The pain you are aware of is in the *anterior deltoid* (front shoulder). This is because the anterior deltoid has been irritated, via reflex nerves, by the *teres minor* (on the outside edge of the shoulder blades) and the lower portion of the *infraspinatus* (attached to the back of the shoulder blades), as shown in Figure 4.18. When you probe the anterior deltoid on someone who has been diagnosed with a "torn rotator cuff," it will be quite painful, but when you press into the teres minor and infraspinatus, they'll hit the roof.

People with teres minor spasticity are also likely to develop pain in the long head of the triceps, which crosses the teres minor and runs down the back of the arm to the elbow. The teres minor is also the main culprit in cases of chronic shoulder dislocation. This is not the result of a muscle being "stretched." It is caused by overly contracted muscles shutting down and letting go in reaction to pain.

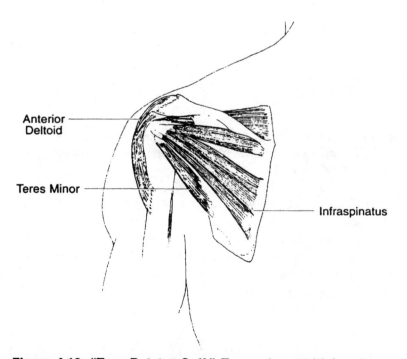

Figure 4.18. "Torn Rotator Cuff." Teres minor and infraspinatus spasticity causes pain in the shoulder that is often misdiagnosed as torn rotator cuff.

Tennis Elbow

Tennis elbow is a painful and sometimes disabling inflammation of the elbow muscles and tissues as a result of grip-
ping something too tightly for too long. Holding a raquet
too tightly, as amateurs often do, is the reason weekend
tennis players are most prone to tennis elbow. Drivers who
habitually hold the steering wheel in a "death grip" may
also suffer from this condition.

Contrary to popular belief, however, tennis elbow has
nothing to do with the elbow joint itself. Whenever you
close your hand tightly around anything, both the *extensor*
and the *flexor* muscles of the forearm come into play. They
are pictured in Figure 4.19. Pain on the outside of the

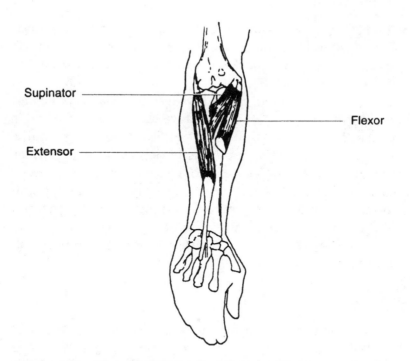

Figure 4.19. "Tennis Elbow." Contrary to what its name implies,
tennis elbow is not a disorder of the elbow joint. Rather, it is the result
of spastic extensor, supinator, and/or flexor muscles of the forearm.

elbow, which is most common, is caused by spasticity in the extensor muscle to the middle finger, which attaches to the outside of your arm. Pain on the inside of the elbow is caused by spasticity in the flexor muscles, which attach to the inside of the arm. A third type of tennis elbow causes pain when you twist your arm from forehand to backhand. This happens when the *supinator* muscle, which crosses from the inside of the elbow to the arm bone, becomes spastic.

At the elbow, the finger muscle attachments make contact with the biceps, triceps, and brachialis muscle attachments of the upper arm and can often spread pain right up the arm to the shoulder or down the arm into the fingers.

Tilted Pelvis

Some people, including most dancers, have a tilted pelvis. This exaggerated lumbosacral angle is often mistaken for swayback. But swayback is a rare congenital deformity of the lower back.

Although a tilted pelvis involves the *gluteus minimus*, this extreme degree of spasm does not occur as a normal part of the basic skewed-torso pattern. You have to really overwork the gluteus minimus to have a tilted pelvis, as seen in Figure 4.20. Dancers do it when they use this muscle to pull their kneecaps up to their noses. This type of movement shortens the muscle so much, it pulls the front of the pelvis down, rotating the buttocks upward. It also increases the stress on the muscles at the lumbosacral joint.

Scoliosis

Scoliosis is a curvature of the spinal column. There two types: lateral and rotary. Both are caused by muscle.

Rotary scoliosis is caused by spasticity in the entire chain of the rotatores and overlying multifidus muscles.

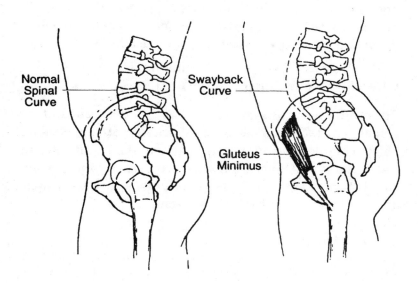

Figure 4.20. Tilted Pelvis. A tilted pelvis, sometimes misdiagnosed as swayback, can result from a spastic gluteus minimus. In a true case of swayback, the front of the spine would follow the dashed line.

These muscles are located on either side of the spinus process, in the center of the back.

Lateral scoliosis—a sideways curvature of the spine—is caused by spastic *spinalis* and *semispinalis* muscles, which overlie the multifidus.

Since doctors generally think that muscles have nothing to do with scoliosis, their cure is to attack the body's skeletal structure. They take steel rods, hook them onto the transverse process (protrusions of bone on the side of the vertebral column) and jack the spine into position. Then they lock the spine in place and leave the rods in. I've seen people who have had the rods snap off when the muscles that caused the original scoliosis grew even more spastic as a result of surgery.

Correcting scoliosis can be accomplished by releasing spasm. However, the amount of time it takes depends on how long the condition has existed. In a teenager, scoliosis may be corrected in a matter of months. In an older adult, it can take years of slow, steady—yet visible—progress.

Central Nervous System Trauma

The central nervous system, consisting of the brain and the spinal chord, coordinates muscle activity. Stroke, cerebral palsy, paraplegia, and quadriplegia are the results of central nervous system trauma, each occuring at different levels of the system. All of these conditions involve muscle and can be treated by releasing spasm.

Cerebral Palsy

Cerebral palsy usually results from a birth trauma to the brain stem. The British more accurately call this condition *cerebellar* palsy, because it actually affects the function of the cerebellum, not the cerebrum. Normally, the cerebellum works through the *reticular nuclei* of the brain stem to control muscle tone. In order for the muscles to perform conscious movements at the request of the cerebrum, the cerebellum has to order the muscles to relax muscle tone. In a person with cerebral palsy, the signal from the cerebellum to the muscles is blocked. Messages from the cerebrum instructing the muscles to move mix with messages from the cerebellum instructing the muscles to remain contracted. That's what causes the characteristic athetoid, or snake-like, movement of someone with cerebral palsy.

In most cases of cerebral palsy, nerves are not damaged. Usually, spasm in the neck muscles, caused by the birth trauma, maintains the disturbance to the brain stem. When the neck muscles which have been affected—the semispinalis cervicis, semispinalis capitis, longus capitis, longus cervicis, splenius cervicis, and splenius capitis—are massaged, the brain stem will correct itself to a very large extent. Massage also needs to be administered to muscles which have become spastic as a result of their struggle to override the blocking action of the cerebellum. These include the suboccipital muscles at the base of the skull, an important group of muscles that we will consider in Chapter 5.

Paraplegia

Paraplegia is paralysis of the lower half of the body. It is caused by extreme trauma to the lower portion of the spinal cord. Following the initial injury, the tissues inside the affected area of the spinal column swell and there is an intense, unremitting firing of nerve impulses. As a result, the muscles contract intensely and become saturated with lactic acid. The brain then receives extremely weak signals from the muscle feedback nerves and instructs the muscles to contract even more. Essentially, paraplegic muscle spasm is no different from other chronic spasm—except in degree.

It is commonly believed that in paraplegia the nerves have been so damaged that they can no longer communicate with muscles. It's true that when the spinal cord actually has been severed, the muscles become limp and flaccid and will atrophy completely. In that case, no treatment can restore them. Much more often, however, paralysis is the result of spastic muscles. In many paraplegics, the muscles become hard, dense, and compacted—a condition that could not possibly exist if the nerves had been severed. The very fact that muscles are contracted to such an extreme degree means that a nerve signal is getting through. The problem is *not* muscle atrophy—but its opposite. The muscle is functioning to an extreme degree. Many doctors and physical therapists, however, do not know how to properly investigate these muscles, and often mistake a shrunken, contracted muscle for one that is no longer functional.

The vast majority of paraplegics are capable of regaining the use of their muscles. Among some four dozen clients with paralysis that I have seen, only one actually had nonfunctional muscles. The others suffered from muscle spasm.

The technique for correcting spasm-induced paraplegia is almost exactly the same as the technique for correcting any other spasticity. The only difference is that, since the muscles are extremely hard and the feedback nerves are severely sickened, it takes much more time to release. The results are usually slow—but steady. The paraplegic's sensitivity to touch is slowly restored, reflexes begin to return, and eventually muscles regain the ability to function.

In addition to massage, I also recommend the use of the Flowtron Intermittent Pressure Garment for treating spasm-induced paraplegia. This device fits around the calf, and simulates the action of walking by squeezing one calf muscle at a time. This pumps the tibial veins and prevents many problems involving poor circulation, including pressure sores and kidney failure—one of the most serious problems for people in wheelchairs.

Quadriplegia

Quadriplegia is paralysis of the entire body below the neck, caused by trauma to the spinal cord in the lower part of the neck.

It is important to understand that in quadriplegia the nerves have not been severed. If a quadriplegic's nerves were severed, the person would be dead. The muscles are not shut down. Rather, as described in the section on paraplegia, they are turned on to the extreme.

Correcting quadriplegia is similar to correcting paraplegia. There is only one difference. Because the injury is so close to the suboccipital muscles which affect metabolism (and are discussed in Chapter 5), quadriplegics also tend to have metabolic problems. These usually are manifested as spiking fevers immediately after the trauma and the inability to maintain normal body weight. This is why most quadriplegics suffer dramatic weight loss, and can even waste away. Paraplegics, on the other hand, frequently gain weight unless they adjust their diet for reduced activity.

Several years ago, I treated a stunt woman who had become quadriplegic after an accident on a film set. Six weeks after the initial trauma, she was still having spiking fevers that ran as high as 106° or 107°F. But one day after I treated her, her fevers subsided.

Stroke

Stroke, a focused trauma that occurs in the cerebrum, cerebellum, or midbrain, tends to affect one side of the body.

The mildest type of stroke takes place when a branch of the carotid artery (the main supply of blood to the head, located in the neck) goes into temporary spasm, decreasing the blood supply to the head. The spasm generally passes within days, sometimes even after a few minutes.

The most traumatic form of stroke, a form that is often fatal, occurs when a blood vessel in the brain bursts. This is usually the result of an aneurysm—the ballooning of an artery wall. Its origin is often genetic.

The most common stroke, however, is the result of a blood clot in one of the small arterioles, or artery branches in the brain. In shutting off blood flow, a clot usually kills off a minimal amount of tissue. However, when cells die, they emit toxins that irritate the nervous system and cause the paralysis associated with stroke. But the muscles affected are actually frozen, not paralyzed. Within six weeks, the immobile muscles often return to a functional state without any treatment at all. Sometimes, however, people don't recover fully. A foot will drag, an arm will not relax, or a hand will not move properly. This happens when the stroke aggravates previously existing spastic conditions.

Massaging frozen muscles to release spasm helps victims of this most common type of stroke to regain mobility.

The conditions we've looked at so far are directly caused by muscle spasm. But the role muscle plays in health gets even more interesting—and surprising—as you'll soon see in the next chapter on the subocipital muscles.

5
The Suboccipital
Muscles

*T*he *suboccipital* muscles are in many ways the most fascinating of all muscle groups, because they are linked to a great number of illnesses and conditions that are never associated with muscle. These tiny muscles at the base of the skull are the key to controlling a vast range of symptoms from allergies and depression to schizophrenia and diabetes. In this chapter, I'll explain exactly why this small group of muscles has such an astonishing impact on both your mental and physical health.

HOW THE SUBOCCIPITAL MUSCLES
BECOME SPASTIC

The iliocostalis, that long muscle responsible for so many middle and lower back problems, is the culprit again—this time for making the suboccipital muscles spastic. The upper portion of the iliocostalis irritates the semispinalis capitis, spreading spasticity from the shoulders up into the suboccipitals. The semispinalis capitis attaches at the C7 transverse, which is a little like Grand Central Station. Five muscles all meet there and irritate each other. The result is a hard knot of spastic muscle I call the "gnaw bone" because when it's massaged, it sounds like a dog gnawing a bone.

This extremely irritable knot spreads spasticity to the suboccipital muscles at the base of the skull, as shown in Figure 5.1. Remember the basic skewed-torso pattern I discussed in the last chapter? It applies here as well. If your torso is pulled to the left, your left suboccipitals will be more spastic than the right. If you're pulled to the right, then your right suboccipitals will be worse.

One of the suboccipital muscles, the *rectus capitis posterior major*, sits right on top of the *greater occipital nerve*. This is one of the most important things you'll ever learn about your body because the greater occipital nerve reflexes to, and therefore influences, the lining of the sphenoid sinus—an organ whose importance to health is nothing short of extraordinary.

THE SPHENOID SINUS

The sphenoid sinus has a powerful effect on the pituitary and the hypothalamus, two extremely important glands located in the brain. Together, these glands control the entire autonomic nervous system, which includes the neuroendocrine system—in other words, they control all of your body chemistry!

The pituitary gland, which is actually an extension of the hypothalamus, must operate at a slightly lower temperature than the rest of the brain. The primary job of the sphenoid sinus is to cool the pituitary. It does this by secreting a clear, serous fluid, which evaporates and cools the sinus cavity (see Figure 5.2).

One of the factors affecting the sphenoid sinus is weather. The sinus linings react continuously to changes in humidity and pressure, which affect the rate at which the serous fluid evaporates. When the humidity and air pressure are low, the sinus membranes tend to sponge up fluid and swell. The pressure changes of airplane travel can also

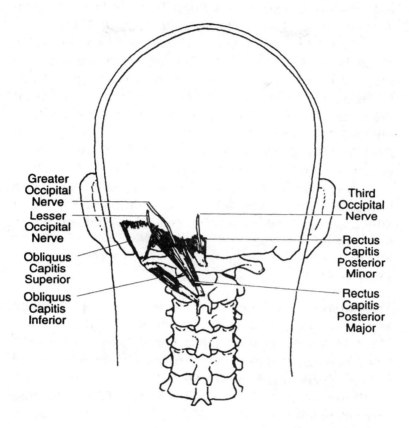

Greater
Occipital
Nerve

Lesser
Occipital
Nerve

Obliquus
Capitis
Superior

Obliquus
Capitis
Inferior

Third
Occipital
Nerve

Rectus
Capitis
Posterior
Minor

Rectus
Capitis
Posterior
Major

Figure 5.1. The Suboccipital Muscles and The Nerves They Irritate.

play havoc with your sinus. In addition, when a spastic rectus capitis posterior major irritates the sphenoid sinus reflex nerve, histamine may be released, stimulating the sinus linings to overproduce fluid. The swollen membranes around the sinus openings then swell shut, and pressure builds up inside the sinus. Doctors seem to be unaware of this. They recognize a blocked sinus only when they see a cloudy picture on an x-ray, indicating pus caused by an infection. They don't realize that sinus cavities can be impacted with clear, serous fluid. This won't show up on an x-ray, but you will certainly suffer from its effects.

When the sphenoid sinus becomes blocked, it loses its ability to cool the pituitary and the hypothalamus. The result may be serious dysfunction of these glands. A blocked and swollen sphenoid sinus can also swell against the bone that separates it from the pituitary, as shown in Figure 5.2. This bone can then press into the pituitary and the bottom of the hypothalamus, affecting the function of your autonomic nervous system.

An irritated or impacted sinus will also cause an excess of histamine to be released. This is an important factor in all kinds of inflammations, from common cold symptoms to outbreaks of herpes.

HISTAMINE

The purpose of histamine is to act as an antiseptic, killing any harmful organisms that invade the body. Histamine also causes inflammation, which is necessary to repair any tissue damage. It is released by *mast cells*, which are found in every part of the body.

When you have a cold or the flu, you get a runny nose and aching joints. These are not caused directly by the cold virus, but by an overproduction of histamine. When you twist an ankle, histamine makes it swell so it can heal.

However, when the sphenoid sinus is irritated, histamine is released when the body does not need it. This produces inflammation, irritation, and symptoms that range from allergies to irritable depression. Excess histamine also aggravates many existing illnesses.

In Short

Because of their relationship to the sphenoid sinus, the suboccipital muscles can be used to relieve any symptoms created by the excess production of histamine. Even more

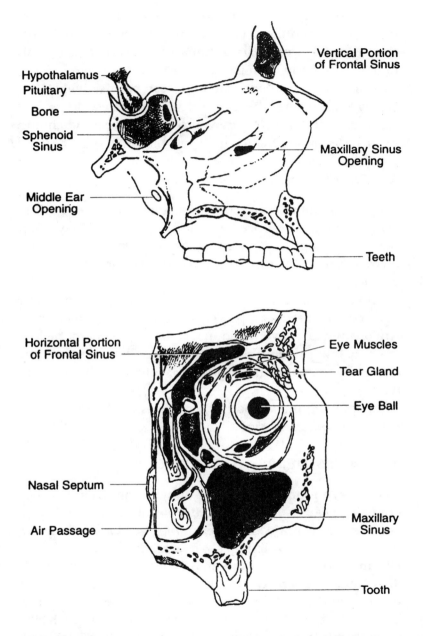

Figure 5.2. The Sphenoid Sinus. The sphenoid sinus has a major impact on health because of its influence on the hypothalamus and pituitary glands.

remarkably—due to the influence of the sphenoid sinus on the pituitary and the hypothalamus—the suboccipital muscles are the key to healing many illnesses involving malfunctions in body chemistry.

All of the conditions that follow can be effectively treated by massaging the suboccipital muscles. In a few instances, other muscles may also be involved and should be included in the treatment.

AGITATED DEPRESSION

People with an irritable sphenoid sinus can suffer terribly from histamine-produced agitated depression. They often seek psychological counselling, but this does little to help them because their problem is not psychological—it is physical.

If you suffer from this type of depression, you may find that the weather has a powerful effect on your emotions. Anyone who has ever lived in California knows that when the dry, low pressure Santa Ana Winds blow, people get extremely irritable—crime goes up, couples fight, tempers flare.

Massaging the suboccipital muscles can provide relief from agitated depression.

ALLERGIES, HERPES, AND HIVES

Allergic symptoms are brought on when an irritable sphenoid sinus causes the overproduction of histamine. If you are allergic to seafood, for example, the iodine released from the seafood irritates an already irritable sinus. Histamine is released and makes your throat inflamed, itchy, and swollen. It can also produce hives. Ruth, the woman in Chapter 1 who was allergic to paper, had impacted sinuses. Irritation produced an excess of histamine in her fingers which made them swell, blister, and peel.

People who have contracted the herpes virus usually experience an outbreak any time conditions irritate the sinuses to cause an overproduction of histamine. One of the reasons women with herpes often have an outbreak just before or after their menstrual period is that their sinuses produce increased histamine at that time.

ASTHMA

The suboccipital muscles play an important role in treating asthma, but other muscles are also involved. The cause and treatment of asthma are discussed in Chapter 6.

BEDWETTING

There are a lot of complicated theories on bedwetting, and parents often torture themselves unnecessarily about what psychological problems it might indicate.

Ordinarily, bedwetting is caused by an irritated sphenoid sinus and the release of histamine in the bladder area. A spastic *obturator internus,* a pelvic muscle, can also cause bladder irritation. However, massaging the suboccipital muscles is usually enough to stop a child's bedwetting after just a few treatments.

BRONCHITIS

Bronchitis is the inflammation of the inside lining of the *bronchioles,* air passageways in the lungs. The tendency to develop bronchitis is genetic—but it is histamine that inflames the bronchioles and causes an attack. Incoming air irritates them further, making it very difficult to breathe. That's why people with bronchitis must take short, shallow breaths.

By relaxing the suboccipitals to drain the sphenoid sinus, histamine is reduced, and breathing becomes easy.

COLD HANDS AND FEET

Your hands and feet contain a large number of histamine-releasing mast cells. There's a good reason for this. Hands and feet make so much contact with other surfaces, that they are likely to suffer injuries—and injuries need histamine to heal. However, histamine constricts the veins and blocks circulation.

In addition, hands and feet do not contain capillaries because capillaries could break when you kick or throw something. Instead, they have blood vessels called *anastomoses*, which are stronger than capillaries, but less efficient at providing adequate blood circulation.

This combination of extra histamine and inefficient anastomoses can make for cold hands and feet. Suboccipital massage can help by reducing histamine production.

COMMON COLD

Quite simply, the common cold is a one-day virus that affects the respiratory tract, followed by several days of histamine overreaction.

When you get a cold, histamine kills the virus. But excess histamine remains, causing the mucus linings to swell. So much fluid is produced, it drips into the nasal passages, tickling the linings, making you sneeze. If there is enough excess mucus to trickle down the throat, you will develop a cough. The throat then produces still more mucus for protection, the lining of the nose swells, the air passages close, and you get all stuffed up. Histamine also excites the joints to overproduce lubricating fluid, making them feel stiff and sore.

The more irritated your sphenoid sinus is, the more severe your symptoms will be, and the longer they will last. Massaging the suboccipitals can reduce suffering time.

DRY SKIN AND PREMATURE AGING

If your sphenoid sinus is disturbed, you are likely to have a problem with dry skin, which will eventually cause premature lines and wrinkles. Pressure on the pituitary causes the overproduction of an anti-diuretic hormone. As a result, the body builds up excess fluid, which evaporates through the skin, causing dryness and chapping. This process is similar to what happens when your lips become chapped from licking them too much. A sign of this type of sinus problem is skin that is so dry that it appears white and flaky.

Suboccipital massage can relieve the pressure on the pituitary which causes the problem.

HEADACHES

Tension in the suboccipital muscles can produce four different types of headaches. Each type of headache is caused by the direct contact of the suboccipitals with a nerve.

Frontal and Cluster Headaches

A frontal headache, marked by pain in the forehead, occurs when the rectus capitis posterior major, one of the key muscles in the suboccipital group, irritates the obliquus capitis superior, a muscle located behind the ear. When the obliquus capitis superior impinges on the lesser occipital nerve (see Figure 5.1), it irritates the frontal sinus, making it swell, and causing a frontal headache.

This can also develop into a "cluster" headache over the eye, which is even more painful than a migraine headache. When the occipital nerve has been chronically impinged over a long period of time, the pain is usually numbed by endorphins. However, as the frontal sinus swells, it begins to press against and distort the forehead bones, frequently causing one eyeball to be lower than the other.

Maxillary Headache

When the third occipital nerve, seen in Figure 5.1, is irritated by the semispinalis capitis muscle near the base of the skull, the nerve irritates the lining of the *maxillary sinuses* (Figure 5.2), located between the eye socket and the upper teeth. This causes pain in the jaw, cheekbone, and upper teeth. But since most people have large enough openings in their maxillary sinuses to keep them from swelling shut, maxillary headache is a fairly rare phenomenon.

Migraine Headache

A migraine headache produces severe pain, often on one side of the head. It is sometimes accompanied by nausea and vomiting.

Migraines occur when the suboccipital muscles irritate the greater occipital nerve and the lesser occipital nerve, seen in Figure 5.1. These nerves then cause irritation and swelling in the sphenoid and frontal sinuses. The sphenoid sinus produces the warning symptoms of visual flashes, nausea, and vomiting. The *frontal sinuses* create pain in the temples by pressing into the jaw muscles there.

Tension Headache

Tension headache is pain at the base of the skull. When you have a tension headache, you are feeling the occipital nerves themselves, seen in Figure 5.1, at the point where a muscle is touching them.

NEARSIGHTEDNESS

Pressure from a swollen frontal sinus can bend the bone that forms the roof of the eye socket. This compresses the eye socket and may distort the cornea, making you nearsighted.

Once the cornea is distorted, nearsightedness *cannot* be

corrected by massaging the suboccipital muscles, though it will stop the condition from getting worse.

People interested in permanently improving their vision without undergoing surgery can participate in a therapy called *orthokeratology*. This technique involves wearing specially fitted contact lenses, which, over time, can change the shape of the cornea.

PREMENSTRUAL SYNDROME (PMS)

Those three little letters, PMS, conjure up in most minds a miserable, bloated female, raging with hormonal anger. Though the effects of PMS appear to be primarily emotional, the condition is actually driven by physiological disturbances that are both hormonal and muscular. Let's look at some of the common symptoms of PMS that can be aided by massaging the suboccipital and other muscles.

Cramps

A week or more before a woman's period, her body secretes a hormone called *prostaglandin*, which causes the uterine contractions that bring on menstruation. Unfortunately, prostaglandin causes *all* muscles to contract to some degree, and can create severe tension in the *external oblique* abdominal muscles which lie over the ovaries. This may cause abdominal cramping, or a pain that seems to come from the ovaries. Massaging the external obliques helps to relieve these pains.

Irritability

The muscle tension caused by prostaglandin can also cause the suboccipitals to become tense, irritating the sphenoid sinus. Histamine is then released, giving you agitated, angry histaminic depression on top of muscular tension. If the frontal sinus becomes irritated (see Figure 5.2), headaches may add to the misery. Massaging the suboccipitals can reverse the cycle of irritability.

Bloating

When the sphenoid sinus swells, it creates pressure on the pituitary. The pituitary, in turn, excretes an anti-diuretic hormone that prevents the body from getting rid of excess fluid. This causes premenstrual bloating.

Swollen Breasts

Prostaglandin sometimes irritates the pectoralis and serratus anterior muscles in the chest. These muscles help pump fluids through the lymphatic ducts that drain the breast. When the muscles are spastic, the ducts become blocked and fluid collects, causing the breasts to get swollen and tender.

Milk ducts in the breast can also become blocked as a result of spastic chest muscles. This can lead to *cystic mastitis,* or lumps in the breast. A doctor may advise that these lumps, or "cysts," be removed surgically. The problem is —there aren't any cysts, only impacted milk ducts that can be drained with massage.

If you first relax the pectoralis and serratus anterior to open the lymph ducts, you can work the lymph and milk ducts themselves, and they will soften and drain.

WEIGHT PROBLEMS

If you find it difficult or impossible to lose weight on diets that work for other people, you may have a problem with your sphenoid sinus. Pressure on the pituitary results in the overproduction of anti-diuretic hormone and the underproduction of two hormones that control glucose metabolism—adrenocorticotropic hormone (ACTH) and thyrotropin. The result—you get bloated *and* fat. Massaging the suboccipital muscles can be extremely effective in treating this condition.

METABOLIC AND AUTOIMMUNE DISEASES

The pituitary and hypothalamus, which control your autonomic nervous system, create the chemical imbalances that produce metabolic and autoimmune diseases. Histamine also plays an important role in these diseases by overstimulating organs and disturbing capillary function. Massage of the suboccipital muscles can be a powerfully effective treatment. Yet, since muscles have been so poorly understood by doctors, this remarkable key to healing these diseases has been completely overlooked.

I have successfully treated several cases of each of the autoimmune and metabolic diseases discussed below. My clinical experience in these areas does not constitute a scientific sample of great size, but the results have certainly been powerful enough to warrant further research.

Autoimmune Diseases

An autoimmune disease is an immune response by the body against one of its own cells or tissues. The predisposition to them is 95 percent genetic. Certain inherited molecules attached to an immune cell, called *human leukocyte antigens* (HLA), have been linked to specific autoimmune diseases. However, the primary cause of the onset of the disease and its symptoms is a malfunction of the hypothalamus.

The hypothalamus controls the immune system and the white blood cells that normally fight invading organisms. In autoimmune diseases, the hypothalamus tells the white blood cells, or leukocytes, to attack the body's own tissues. Following are some of the diseases that can be treated with suboccipital massage to restore normal function to the hypothalamus.

Lupus

Lupus is a disease in which white blood cells attack the tis-

sues of the body's organs. Most frequently, this process
starts in the kidneys. If they fail, the blood becomes toxic.

Lupus also causes the production of excess histamine,
which produces skin rashes, usually near the joints, the
cheeks, and the nose. The word lupus is Latin for wolf, and
the disease was so named because the face rash it produces,
or "mask of lupus," resembles patterns seen on certain
breeds of wolf. Lupus can be treated by massaging the suboccipital muscles to correct the hypothalamus and reduce
histamine production.

Multiple Sclerosis

In multiple sclerosis (MS), the white blood cells attack the
fatty *myelin* protective covering of the nerves. Eventually
the nerves weaken and cannot adequately stimulate the
muscles to perform properly. The disease itself may be
brought into remission by working the suboccipital muscles and correcting any hypothalamus malfunction.
Immediate, short-term comfort and increased strength can
also be provided by relaxing the specific muscles affected
by the disease.

Rheumatoid Arthritis

Rheumatoid arthritis is an autoimmune disease in which
the body's white blood cells attack the cartilage of joints,
causing them to become inflamed with fluid. This causes
pain and loss of movement and may sometimes lead to the
destruction of the joint. (This disease should not be confused with osteoarthritis, which is discussed in Chapter 4.)

Doctors often prescribe cortisone to relieve the symptoms associated with rheumatoid arthritis. However, there
are benefits and drawbacks to using this drug. It is effective
in suppressing the immune system, thereby preventing a
white-blood-cell attack on joint cartilage, but it makes you
vulnerable to colds and infections. As an antihistamine (not

Why Women Are More Susceptible to Autoimmune Diseases Than Men

Most of the people who suffer from autoimmune diseases such as multiple sclerosis, rheumatoid arthritis, and lupus are women. That's because, in addition to being autoimmune diseases, they are also collagen diseases. And collagen production in men and women differs. This difference is responsible for the higher risk of autoimmune disease in women.

Collagen is a protein that is crucial for maintaining the structure of every organ of the body. Lack of collagen causes tissue to degenerate. Autoimmune diseases cause a breakdown of collagen in the affected areas.

The collagen supply in men and preadolescent girls is regulated by the adrenal glands. (The adrenals are also supposed to regulate collagen supply in post-menopausal women, but as you'll see in the discussion on osteoporosis, the adrenals often do a poor job of it.) During a woman's reproductive years, collagen regulation is taken over by the ovaries because they are able to produce the enormous amount of collagen required to build a baby's body.

Unfortunately, because the female hormone cycle is a whole symphony of events, the ovaries are far less stable than the adrenal glands. As a result, the ovaries cannot always control collagen production as effectively as the adrenal glands. Therefore, since a woman's body cannot replace the collagen destroyed by the autoimmune reaction as effectively as a man's, women are far more vulnerable to multiple sclerosis, rheumatoid arthritis, and lupus than are men.

In addition, it has been found that, once an immune response has been triggered, female hormones excite the production of elevated quantities of gamma interferon, a substance that accelerates the immune response. This is helpful in combatting an invading organism, and may be one of the reasons women live longer than men. However, in people with the predisposition to an autoimmune disease, gamma interferon can spark an autoimmune reaction.

an anti-inflammatory drug as is generally thought), cortisone can also provide some relief of the inflammation caused by rheumatoid arthritis. But the body responds to the loss of histamine by producing more histamine. The result is an ever-increasing need for the drug. There are also other well-known side effects of cortisone. It turns protein to fat; shrinks muscles; causes fluid retention; and disturbs metabolism, adrenal gland function, and even the heart.

People suffering from rheumatoid arthritis can benefit greatly from two methods of treatment. First, immediate relief can be provided by working the muscles around the affected joint to drain excess fluid. This contradicts the standard medical explanation that swelling is produced by a "rheumatoid factor" (an unidentified substance found in the blood of everyone with the disease) which adheres to channels in the joint lining, preventing fluid from escaping. If this were true, the joint would not drain when the muscles around it were relaxed. Yet I have drained some enormously swollen joints. In a much slower process, working the suboccipital muscles can eventually stop the autoimmune reaction from causing further degeneration to the joints.

Metabolic Diseases

The cause of metabolic diseases such as hypoglycemia, schizophrenia, and manic depression—like autoimmune diseases—is mainly genetic. However, the symptoms of metabolic diseases result from malfunctioning hypothalamus and pituitary glands, which regulate hormones—the body's chemical messengers.

It is now widely recognized that diabetes, schizophrenia, and manic depression are metabolic disorders, and that metabolism is regulated by the hypothalamus and the pituitary. If follows, then, that normalizing hypothalamic and pituitary function by massaging the suboccipital muscles that affect them can correct these diseases.

Autism, Hyperkinesis, and Schizophrenia

Schizophrenia is a metabolic disease, as are its juvenile forms: autism and hyperkinesis.

They all involve a disturbance to the hypothalamus. In schizophrenia, a body chemical affects the sensory nerves, so that a schizophrenic will see, hear, and feel things that are not real. Behavior can run the gamut from catatonia (the inability to move) to hyperambulism (the inability to sit). Autistic children do not react to their environment. They experience delayed speech development, unresponsiveness to love and affection, and behavior that ranges from total silence to periods of hyperactivity. Hyperkinetic (or hyperactive) children suffer from lack of concentration, self-destructiveness, and impatience.

For years schizophrenia was thought to be a mental illness until an experiment proved it to be metabolic. In the experiment, a person experiencing a schizophrenic attack was put on a dialysis machine, which removes dangerous waste products and excess fluids from the bloodstream. The attack stopped. This clearly showed that the cause of a schizophrenic episode had to be a substance that could be removed from the blood.

By relaxing the *suboccipital* muscles and correcting the metabolic disturbance, I have produced dramatic changes in the behavior of schizophrenics and autistic and hyperkinetic children.

Diabetes Mellitus

Diabetes mellitus is a metabolic disease which, in many ways, resembles an autoimmune disease because the immune system attacks and destroys one of its own tissues. (In fact, juvenile diabetes is now classified as an autoimmune disease.) In diabetes, the immune system attacks the islets of Langerhans in the pancreas. This impairs insulin production. Without insulin the body cannot utilize glucose, thus creating a high level of glucose in the blood and a low level of glucose absorption by the tissues.

In the early stages of diabetes, the islets of Langerhans undergo no structural damage. Postmortem studies performed on young diabetics and people in the early stages of the disease who had been killed in automobile accidents found normal, healthy-looking pancreases with no pathology to indicate diabetes. In postmortem studies of older diabetics, however, the islets of Langerhans of the pancreases showed signs of degeneration. Regulating the hypothalamus, which controls immune response, by massaging the suboccipital muscles in the early stages of the disease should prevent the islet of Langerhans from degenerating.

Poor circulation is one of the most serious problems in advanced diabetes, yet high blood sugar levels do not affect circulation. The cause is histamine, which attacks the membranes surrounding capillaries and arterioles.

I have been most successful working with people in the initial stages of diabetes, who were still on the oral medication Orinase. The muscle treatment can be very powerful. In fact, after I administered one treatment to a young diabetic boy, he immediately began to manufacture his own insulin. During the trip home, he went into insulin shock because his body was not used to handling the amount of insulin produced after the treatment.

Epilepsy

An epileptic attack at its most severe can involve convulsions and loss of consciousness. It is similar to a schizophrenic attack, except that it affects the motor nerves instead of the sensory nerves. Just as the schizophrenic sees and hears things that are not there, the epileptic has motor impulses over which he has no control. At one time, epilepsy, like schizophrenia, was considered a mental disease. Now we recognize that epilepsy is metabolic in nature.

A disturbance of the hypothalamus causes a substance

to be produced that triggers epilepsy. The drug Dilantin will block the triggering substance. However, if the epileptic attacks are not due to brain tumors, they can also be prevented by working the suboccipital muscles and restoring the normal function of the hypothalamus.

Hypoglycemia and Chronic Fatigue Syndrome

There are two distinct types of hypoglycemia, an abnormally low level of glucose in the blood. One is a prediabetic insulin hypoglycemia caused by the hypothalamus. The other—and most common form of hypoglycemia—has no relation at all to diabetes. It occurs when the pituitary releases cortical steroids, which are manufactured in the adrenal glands and control blood sugar level. Cortical steroids can cause blood sugar levels to plummet, resulting in weakness and depression.

Chronic fatigue syndrome has several contributing causes. The overproduction of histamine creates an agitated depression, and a metabolic disturbance reduces the strength of the immune system. But the major symptom—an overwhelming feeling of fatigue—is the result of an extreme form of adrenal hypoglycemia.

Treatment of the suboccipital muscles can correct the metabolic imbalance, and restore a person to a healthy, energetic state.

Manic Depression

The extremely high and low mood swings of manic depression are recognized by psychologists and psychiatrists as a metabolic dysfunction. In manic depression, the hypothalamus causes an imbalance of sodium and potassium in the blood. Because of the way this disease affects the kidneys, a person having a manic depressive episode will tend to excrete excessive amounts of potassium in urine.

Lithium, which restores the body's balance of sodium

and potassium, is currently the drug of choice for treating this disease. But lithium has negative side effects, such as fatigue and the loss of concentration. Instead of treating manic depression with lithium, symptoms can be reduced by massaging the suboccipitals and restoring normal function to the hypothalamus.

Osteoporosis

Osteoporosis, most commonly found in post-menopausal women, is a condition in which bones become porous and brittle and are easily fractured. Often, this results in pain, loss of height, and other bone deformities.

Contrary to popular belief, osteoporosis is *not* the result of calcium deficiency. Rather, it is caused by a malfunction of collagen metabolism.

Bone is made up of a matrix scaffold of collagen fibers to which calcium crystals attach. Like all the other tissues of the body, bones are constantly being rebuilt. First, a cell called an *osteoclast* tears down a small section of the bone. Then the collagen matrix is rebuilt by a cell called an *osteoblast*. The matrix generates a negative electric charge, which attracts positively charged calcium crystals that attach themselves to the bone. The osteoclasts carry on their destructive activity with no outside aid, but the osteoblasts must be constantly supplied with new collagen in order to rebuild the collagen matrix. Without adequate collagen to form the collagen matrix, even dense bone can become brittle, like concrete that has not been reinforced.

In a woman's child-bearing years collagen production is controlled by the ovaries. During menopause, the ovaries give up this job and the adrenal glands are supposed to take over—but they must be activated by the pituitary. As you know, the function of the pituitary gland can be compromised when spastic suboccipital muscles irritate the sphenoid sinus. When this happens, the necessary collagen is not supplied. So while the osteoclast continues to eat holes in the bones, the osteoblast cannot rebuild them.

Massaging the suboccipital muscles can restore pituitary function so that the adrenal glands can once again provide collagen to rebuild the bones.

A CALL TO RESEARCH

I never cease to be amazed at all the functions of the body that are influenced by the sphenoid sinus and its effect on both histamine production and the entire autonomic nervous system. By massaging the suboccipital muscles, many illnesses can be brought under control or healed without the use of drugs—and without the damaging side effects that go with them. It is an area that medicine must begin to explore.

6
Muscle and Your Internal Organs

Not only are your sinuses and glands affected by spastic muscles, other internal organs are as well. In addition to the usual ways that spasm spreads—pressure, irritation, and blocked circulation—there's a fourth factor at work—reflex points.

Pain lets you know when an organ is irritated, infected, or injured. But the internal organs are insensate—they do not have nerves to transmit pain. Instead, they have a neurological connection to muscles and communicate pain by touching, or "reflexing," to muscles. Muscles, in turn, send pain signals from the organs to surface nerves. This lets us know when an organ is in trouble—but it also provides another way to develop spasm. An organ inflamed by infection or allergy can irritate a specific muscle and make it spastic. That same spastic muscle may then further irritate the organ.

Let's look now at some conditions that affect the internal organs and see how they are related to muscles.

ANGINA, ATHEROSCLEROSIS, AND HEART ATTACKS

Diseases of the heart kill more Americans than any other illnesses. By far the most prevalent heart problem is *atherosclerosis*, a blockage of the coronary arteries caused by cholesterol plaquing, that can lead to a heart attack. Muscle spasm is a contributing factor to this disease—and also provides a means of healing it that may make the ordeal of bypass surgery unnecessary.

To understand how muscles affect your arteries, you must first understand what makes cholesterol adhere to the artery walls. Most health practitioners place the blame on diet and the amount of cholesterol and saturated fats in the bloodstream. However, as the experiment below clearly shows—while the amount of cholesterol in the blood may eventually become a factor in plaquing—it is *not* the cause.

Scientists fed one group of test animals a high cholesterol diet and another a low cholesterol diet. Neither group developed significant arterial plaquing. They then repeated the experiment—this time using a chemical which caused arterial tension—and *both* groups developed plaquing, though it was worse in the animals with high cholesterol diets. This clearly demonstrated that plaquing starts with irritation to the arteries—not the presence of cholesterol. Once plaquing has begun, however, the amount of cholesterol in the blood becomes significant.

Irritation to the artery walls causes them to spasm and shed cells. These dead cells build up into little mounds that attract and hold cholesterol. In Chapter 3 we mentioned that one cause of spastic artery walls is excess lactic acid in the bloodstream. An even more powerful factor is spasm in the pectoralis major, the pectoralis minor, and the serratus anterior, muscles that reflex to the heart and coronary arteries. During a heart attack, the pain that shoots down the arm to the hand comes from these muscles. When they are spastic, they irritate the arteries, and can cause cholesterol plaquing.

People who are doing aerobic exercise to ward off heart problems should take note of another recent finding. Researchers found, not surprisingly, that if you don't exercise at all, it's bad for your heart, while jogging approximately 5 miles a week can be beneficial. What was startling in this study was the discovery that jogging 10 miles a week is as bad for your heart as doing no exercise at all—and jogging 15 miles a week is actually *worse* than not exercising at all! Remember, moderation in all things.

Once we understand that muscle spasm causes cholesterol plaquing, we can learn to prevent heart attacks. This knowledge is also the key to clearing blocked arteries without bypass surgery because, when you release spasm in the involved muscles, the artery walls become smooth again and the plaqued cholesterol dissolves back into the bloodstream.

I have had several clients who suffered from angina, chest pains associated with an insufficient supply of blood to the heart. A dramatic reduction in attacks occurred when their spastic pectoral muscles were relaxed. The number of people I have worked with in this area may constitute a small sample in scientific terms—but the effects of treatment are too positive to overlook.

ASTHMA

Asthma is a lung disorder marked by attacks of breathing difficulty. The symptoms range from wheezing, coughing, and breathlessness to total inability to breathe. The predisposition to asthma is genetic. However, the symptoms are caused by muscle spasm and the excess production of histamine.

Normally, when a person inhales, the diaphragm muscle pulls downward, causing a partial vacuum in the enclosed rib cage above. This vacuum pulls on the lungs and their air ducts, the bronchioles, as shown in Figure 6.1. The muscles around the bronchioles then contract and stiffen so as not to collapse into the vacuum. At the same

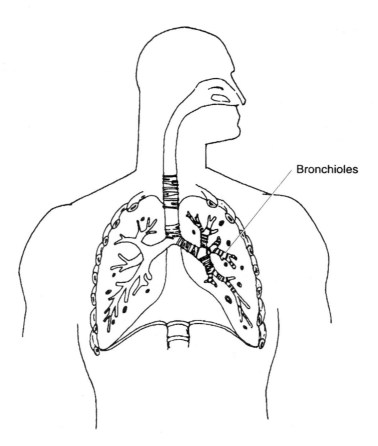

Figure 6.1. Asthma. In an asthmatic, the bronchial muscles remain contracted on the exhale because they are irritated either by spastic trapezius and intercostal muscles or excess histamine production.

time, a round portion of the trapezius (between the mid-back and shoulders) and the associated intercostals (which are reflexively coupled with the diaphragm and bronchial muscles) contract in order to stabilize the vertebrae on which the diaphragm is pulling. In an asthmatic, the bronchial muscles are irritated and tend to remain contracted on the exhale. This restricts the flow of air, causing breathing difficulty.

In addition to this, a factor called an H cell has been identified in people with asthma. H cells are sensitive to histamine. If someone with a predisposition to asthma has a congested sphenoid sinus, the excess histamine produced will cause their H cells to excite the already contracted muscles around the bronchioles even more.

The treatment of asthma involves relaxing the trapezius and intercostal muscles as well as the suboccipital muscles which affect histamine production.

BABY COLIC

Colic, a painful abdominal condition in infants, is caused by a spastic *intertransversarii* muscle. This is a spinal muscle that reflexes to the *pyloric sphincter,* a muscular ring that separates the stomach from the first part of the small intestine.

I've had the opportunity to work on infants as young as one week old. The intertransversarii muscles were stiff, indicating that spasm had been forming for several months. After treatment there was no more colic.

HIGH BLOOD PRESSURE

Blood pressure can become abnormally and dangerously elevated for several reasons. Spastic muscle is one. The carotid artery is a major blood vessel that brings blood to the head and neck. Applying finger pressure above the *carotid body*, a pressure point on the artery, will make blood pressure decrease. Applying pressure below the carotid body makes blood pressure increase. The sternocleidomastoid is positioned along the carotid body. When the sternocleidomastoid is spastic, it can make blood pressure rise or fall just as applying finger pressure would. Releasing spasticity in this muscle can help to normalize some types of high blood pressure.

Kidney function may also influence blood pressure. For

proper filtration of waste to occur in the kidneys, a minimum level of blood pressure needs to be maintained in kidney blood vessels. But circulation in the kidneys can become impaired by a spastic iliocostalis. If this happens, blood pressure rises to accommodate kidney filtration. Releasing spasm in the iliocostalis can help correct high blood pressure related to kidney function.

INTESTINAL AND STOMACH PROBLEMS

To understand many intestinal and stomach problems, we have to refer to the basic skewed-torso pattern of spasticity. This is because people who are pulled to the left will have symptoms that are completely different from those who are pulled to the right.

Body Pulled to the Left

When your body is pulled to the left, you are more likely to be constipated and suffer from colitis and heartburn. Let's examine the reasons for this.

If the psoas and the external oblique muscles on your left side are spastic, as shown in Figure 6.2, they can press against the sigmoid portion of the descending colon, restricting the passage of feces, and causing constipation. Constant irritation of the colon by spastic muscles may also cause colitis—inflammation of the colon. And if restriction of the colon causes gas pressure to build up, diverticulitis—a ballooning of the colon wall—can result.

Heartburn is caused by a spastic intertransversarii muscle. The intertransversarii muscle at the third lumbar vertebra on your left side reflexes to the *cardiac sphincter*—the inlet valve into the stomach—and can cause you to belch-up partially digested food or have trouble swallowing if the muscle is overly contracted. The cardiac sphincter, named for its location near the heart, has nothing to do with the heart, but gives us the term heartburn.

Body Pulled to the Right

If your body is pulled to the right, you'll tend to have gas, a soft bowel movement, and ulcers.

On your right side, the quadratus lumborum to the third lumbar vertebra can produce spasm in the adjacent inter-transversarii muscle. The intertransversarii reflexes to the pyloric sphincter, the outlet valve of the stomach. If the pyloric sphincter muscle is irritated by a spastic intertrans-versarii, the sphincter contracts and produces more lactic acid than usual. The veins responsible for removing the lactic acid from the sphincter become overloaded. Excess lactic acid seeps into the surrounding tissues, causing the mast cells in those tissue to release histamine. The histamine excites the stomach to produce excess hydrochloric acid. When this happens, you may feel hungry all the time. People who like to constantly nibble, or "graze," usually have this problem. The stomach irritation also causes gastric mucus to be produced. This protects the stomach lining. Unfortunately, some people host a bacteria that destroys the mucus. When there is too much acid and not enough mucus, ulcers may develop. Excess hydrochloric acid can also cause a tendency to belch after eating certain foods. If an irritated sphenoid sinus is also causing an overproduction of histamine, these stomach problems can be more acute.

Soft bowel movements, diarrhea, gurgling, and intestinal gas are conditions attributable to spasm in the abdominal external oblique and the underlying psoas on your right side. Here's why. The external oblique sits over the *ileocecal valve*, as shown in Figure 6.2. The ileocecal valve permits the contents of the small intestine to flow into the large intestine in a forward direction only. But if the oblique and psoas are both spastic, they can trap the valve and increase the pressure required to open it. The increased pressure supplied by intestinal gas then pushes through the valve so energetically, it carries unintended fluid into the colon. This results in soft bowel movements, diarrhea, intestinal gurgling, and gas.

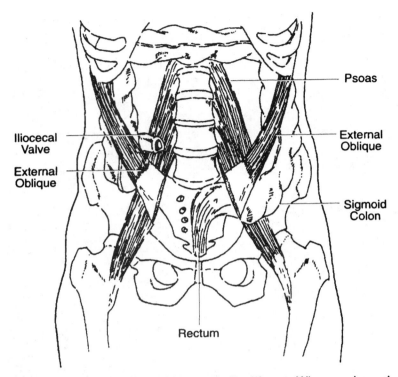

Psoas

External
Oblique

Sigmoid
Colon

Iliocecal
Valve

External
Oblique

Rectum

Figure 6.2. Intestinal and Stomach Problems. When a skewed
torso pulls your body to the left, spastic oblique and psoas muscles
on your left side press against the sigmoid colon, leading to constipation, colitis, and diverticulitis. When your body is pulled to the right,
spastic external oblique and psoas muscles on your right side trap
the ileocecal valve, leading to intestinal gurgling, diarrhea, and gas.

KIDNEY PROBLEMS

Spastic muscle is not the cause of most kidney diseases. But
it can cause existing kidney conditions, such as malfunctioning kidneys and kidney stones, to last much longer
than they should.

The portion of the iliocostalis muscle between the
pelvis and the ribs reflexes to the kidneys. This is the area
of pain associated with kidney infection. When the spastic-

ity in this section of the iliocostalis is strong enough, it may interfere with kidney function. Constant reflex irritation from the iliocostalis can disturb the temperature of the kidney and may be a factor in producing kidney stones.

Releasing spasm in the iliocostalis stops the reflex irritation to the kidneys. In several cases, I have been able to restore kidney function to clients who had suffered from malfunctioning kidneys.

PELVIC ORGAN PROBLEMS

Important organs in the pelvic area include the bladder, the anal sphincter, the sexual organs, the uterus in women, and the prostate in men. When spastic, two muscles—the *obturator internus* and the *pyramidalis*—may cause problems in these areas.

The obturator internus wraps around the lower portion of the pelvis, then extends out and attaches to the leg bone. Every time you take a step and your muscles contract and relax, the obturator internus acts as a circulatory sump pump, pumping the blood up and out of this body cavity. By impinging on veins in the pelvic area, a spastic obturator internus can reduce blood flow and lead to such problems as hemorrhoids, uterine problems, an enlarged prostate, impotence and frigidity, an irritable bladder, and bladder infections. It can also aggravate infections and other existing conditions.

The pyramidalis muscle, located at the middle of the pubic bone, is directly connected to the bladder. When spastic, the pyramidalis can contribute to an irritable bladder, as well as to some prostate or uterus problems.

HEALING YOUR BODY

Up to this point, I've been focusing on what's wrong with you. In Part 3, I'll tell you how you can set things right again!

PART THREE

How You
Can Be Helped

Part 1 of this book introduced you to hypertonic muscle spasm and its influence on your health, and Part 2 detailed the many conditions that result from spasm. Now, in Part 3, it's time to learn what can be done to rid the body of spasm and return it to good health.

Chapter 7 describes the massage that will release muscle spasm. This technique took years to develop, and it takes quite some time to master—but it works! Finally, Chapter 8 tells you how you can exercise—and keep your body healthy and spasm-free.

7

The Neuromuscular
Massage Treatment

*T*his chapter will provide an understanding of the neuromuscular therapy I've developed to release muscle spasm and return the body to health. For the lay person, it will explain the principles and techniques involved in this unique treatment. For the health care professional, it's the starting point for learning a powerful new method of therapy.

However, I cannot stress enough that simply reading this chapter will *not* enable you to begin using this technique. You can't even learn it in a crash course or with a few weeks of practice because it requires not only a thorough knowledge of physiology, but manual proficiency and clinical skill that can only be acquired with time.

LEARNING THE TECHNIQUE

Learning this massage is like learning to play the violin. You can read an instruction manual or have a teacher show you exactly how to hold the violin, where to place your fingers on the strings, and how to stroke the bow. But you will not be able to play. Mentally, you may know exactly what to do, but your hands will still be ignorant.

As time allows, I train a few people in this work. In the process, I am learning the ins and outs of how to teach. One of the reasons it takes a while to learn these techniques is that mastery isn't entirely under the student's conscious control. Part of the learning process takes place in the cerebellum, or unconscious mind. A piano player with amnesia, who can't remember ever having taken piano lessons, can still play the piano. That's because the cerebellum remembers even when the cerebrum—the conscious mind—does not. In order to learn neuromuscular massage, a connection must be made between these two parts of the brain. It's always fascinating to watch students when they start out. It looks as if they're never going to get it, and then suddenly, one day, the link is made. And that unconscious connection is just the first step. Learning this neuromuscular technique requires years of study—and practice, practice, practice.

Whenever anyone comes to me wanting to learn this work, I show them two porcelain bowls in my office. Working with porcelain requires much greater care than working with clay. If you apply too little pressure to the porcelain, it won't reach the point at which it becomes plastic and begins to flow. If you apply too much pressure, the porcelain will become fluid and runny, so you must maintain just the right pressure at all times. What makes this even more difficult is that the water in the porcelain mixture is always evaporating, so the plasticity point is constantly changing and can be understood only by a very perceptive sense of touch.

The first porcelain bowl was made by one of my students before she began training with me. You can tell it's a good piece work because of the way light occasionally shows through it. She made the second bowl after she'd been working with muscle for nine months. It is an extraordinary piece of work, and so translucent that it seems illuminated from within. Your fingers must develop this same level of skill before you can effectively do neuromuscular massage.

Now that you realize you can't just read this chapter and go to work, I can give you an idea of what is involved in releasing spasm.

WHAT REALLY NEEDS HEALING?

In order to know what neuromuscular massage must accomplish, we first have to identify exactly what needs to be healed.

The muscle itself does not need healing. A muscle contracted in chronic spasm is not only functioning, it is working above and beyond normal requirements. So our purpose is not to overpower the muscle, because the *muscle* is not the source of the problem.

Similarly, the circulatory system is not to blame for muscle spasm. Although hypertonic muscle blocks circulation, the circulatory system is designed to be compressed by muscle—that's how blood is pumped back to the heart. While compressed veins do keep lactic acid trapped in the muscle, there's nothing actually wrong with the blood vessels themselves. So that is not where we direct our attack.

Even the nerves that send signals *from* the brain to the muscle are not to blame for spasm. Since spastic muscle is overly-contracted muscle, the nerve signal from the brain is coming through loud and clear.

The only part of this system that is actually malfunctioning is the feedback nerves. As you read in Chapter 3, the feedback nerves tell the brain whether a muscle needs to be tightened or relaxed to maintain muscle tone. When lactic acid sickens the feedback nerves, they send a weakened signal to the brain. The brain, receiving the weak signal, thinks the muscle is too relaxed and commands it to tighten. This is how spasm develops. The cause of the problem is lactic acid, but it can't be dealt with directly. It is being squeezed into the muscle, but there is no way it can be squeezed out on its own. The signal of the feedback nerves to the brain must be increased, so that the brain will command the muscle to release.

The main goal in this massage feedback is to stimulate and heal the feedback nerves without activating the anulospiral nerves that control the stretch reflex. If the massage is done correctly, the muscle will relax, the blood vessels will open, lactic acid will be carried away to the liver, and the muscle will return to a state of health.

Now let's take a look at how it's done.

WORKING THE PATTERN

The first thing you have to do is to identify the muscles that are tight. With the person lying down on a massage table or bed, roll your fingers across—not along—the muscles and notice which fibers do not give. Once you find the areas of tightness, you need a thorough knowledge of the pattern of spasticity—the crucial interrelationship of muscles described in Chapter 4—in order to work the body effectively. In most cases, a symptom is part of an overall pattern of spasticity, and correcting it requires working the whole pattern, not just one isolated area. I began to realize this early in my practice. I would be working on a knot in the shoulder, and the lower back would suddenly ease up. A common mistake people make when trying to relieve symptoms with massage is to work only in the area of pain.

LAYERS OF SPASTICITY

Round muscle forms spasm in layers. These are not layers of muscle fibers. Rather, they are what you might call layers of trauma. These cylindrical layers have been built up over the years by a succession of irritation, and they actually represent different points in time. In some ways, working a muscle in spasm is like an archaeological dig. When you go down into the muscle, relaxing layer after layer, you are also going back to the time they were created. Sometimes, when you release a layer that had an emotional coupling—that is, when emotional and physical trauma were simultaneous—the person may react exactly as he or she had at that earlier time.

There is a tendency for a given layer, regardless of thickness, to release as a whole. It is impossible to predict and control when this release will occur. Sometimes more than one layer will release in a session. Sometimes none will. But even when you don't see an immediate result from your efforts, you have still accomplished something because you are stimulating the feedback nerves, and the effect is cumulative.

For some clients, symptoms disappear after only one or two sessions. This occurs when only the outer layers of spastic muscle are involved. With others, I can work for a long time, going deeper and deeper, making the knot of spasticity smaller and smaller, yet there seems to be no change. Sometimes the nerve irritation persists until the last inevitable minute, and then, suddenly, the involved muscle releases.

A television actor who was nearly fifty years old started treatment with me at the same time as a thirteen-year-old soccer player. They both had the same skewed-torso problem, except that the actor's torso was pulled over much farther than the boy's. The actor was working on a film in downtown Los Angeles in the heat of summer, and had to wear a jacket to hide his distortion. Generally, the older person has the longer-standing condition and takes longer to respond to treatment. But in this case, the actor straightened up with the first treatment, while the thirteen-year-old showed no response at all. The boy had been playing soccer since he was five or six, which meant that he'd been taking quite a beating for some time. In fact, in a photo he showed me, he was up in the air kicking a soccer ball while another boy was kicking him. Week after week, month after month, the boy's mother brought him in, but the muscles just wouldn't budge. Finally, after nine months, while he was on the table, one leg suddenly dropped down and was even with the other.

Each body releases spasm in its own time. While the patterns of spasticity are alike, every person is a unique variation on the theme.

THE MASSAGE TECHNIQUE

- **Rule 1.** *Use only the fingers to massage.* This work requires enormous precision. That's why it's done with the index and the middle fingers only—not the palms, or the elbows, or the flat of the hand. The tips of the fingers are too hard, and the balls are too soft. The place in between is just right. In order to keep the right part of your fingertip in contact with the muscle, the angle of your finger to your palm should be 30 degrees as should the angle of your palm to your forearm, as shown in Figure 7.1.

- **Rule 2.** *Maintain pressure as close as possible to the stretch-reflex point without activating the stretch reflex.* When exerting pressure on the muscle, you must go to the point just before the stretch reflex turns on without going past it. When you press on a muscle, lightly increasing the pressure, it will soon begin to resist. After a certain point, you will feel it go from soft and flexible, to hard and tight, almost like you've hit bottom. You've just over-stimulated the anulospiral nerves and turned on the stretch reflex. Now the muscle is contracted, and you are making the spasm worse, not better. But if you work too lightly, staying too far back from the stretch-reflex point, you will not provide enough stimulation to the feedback nerves. You've got to hang right on that line. This is knowledge that your fingers can acquire only with experience. The more you practice, the smarter your hands will become.

- **Rule 3:** *Stroke as fast as possible without activating the stretch* *reflex.* The feedback nerves respond to speed as well as pressure. The more rapidly a change occurs in the muscle, the greater the nerve output. This is why you want to stroke as fast as possible. But when you are first learning this massage technique, you will have to sacrifice speed for sensitivity, so that you can remain aware of the stretch reflex point. Speed will only come with time.

- **Rule 4**: *Stroke across the grain of the muscle instead of along it.* Stroking along the grain activates the stretch reflex. Instead, stroke across the grain by making your fingers follow the contour of the muscle—up, over, and down. As you work across the grain of the muscle, you will have to change the angle of your fingers to your palm and the angle of your palm to your forearm to keep the right part of your fingertip in contact with the muscle. Do not drag your fingers through the muscle. This can activate the stretch reflex. When working without oil, you'll have to take the skin with you over to the other side of the muscle as you stroke forward, then carry the skin back with almost no pressure. This requires tremendous coordination because you must maintain proper pressure and finger angle at all times. With time and practice, your hands will learn to do this automatically.

- **Rule 5**: *Use long strokes.* The hard core of spastic muscle is usually so irritable that it can take very little pressure. Therefore, each massage stroke must be long enough to take you across the entire muscle, not just the hard core. Long strokes distribute pressure evenly throughout the muscle, providing enough stimulation to be beneficial without causing a stretch-reflex reaction.

- **Rule 6**: *Do not stroke too many times in one place.* After you work a muscle for a certain amount of time, it stops responding. Experience will teach you to feel when this happens, but the beginner will not be able to tell. For this reason, it's important not to stroke too many times in one

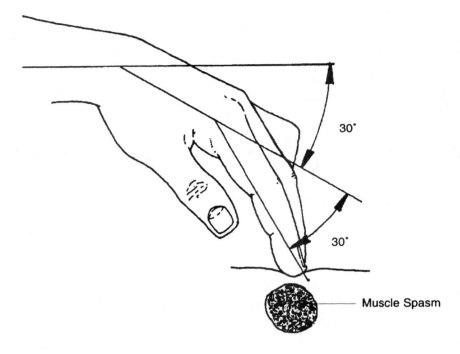

30°

30°

Muscle Spasm

Figure 7.1. The Massage Technique.

place. Administer six strokes to one area, move to a different area, and come back later.

- **Rule 7**: *Use oil in the beginning.* I work without oil because it's simple and there's no mess. But when you are first starting out, it's a good idea to use oil because it will help promote long strokes and your fingers will slide across the skin instead of carrying it along. What kind of oil should you use? Any massage oil will do. How much should you use? If your subject slides off the table, you've used too much.

- **Rule 8**: *Alternately stroke and percuss the muscle.* Stroking involves distributing light pressure over an area. It provides broad surface stimulation to the muscle. Percussive movement, sometimes called *topoment*, is an intense, concentrated, controlled tapping of the muscle. The percussion must be very short and very fast. There is a fraction-of-a-second delay in the stretch-reflex response, and because of this you can use considerably more pressure with percussing than with stroking. This allows you to work on deep tissues you could not otherwise reach.

The Bio-Pulser Option

Like the stroking technique, the percussive technique takes a long time to perfect, so I've designed a machine to eliminate the need to learn it.

My machine is called the Bio-Pulser, and it percusses faster than is humanly possible. Unlike commercial vibrators, it is not driven by a simple crank that mindlessly thumps. Instead, it has a cam programmed to produce a thrust that will generate strong biological nerve response. With other massagers, even those with a percussive movement, each thrust takes too long, and there are too many thrusts per second. This overloads the nerve circuits and produces a jumbled, tingling response which does nothing to release spasm. The Bio-Pulser provides fewer thrusts per second, and each thrust is of extremely short duration. It has been carefully designed to be compatible with the biological recovery period of the nerve circuits, so that your nervous system can integrate the stimulation. The Bio-Pulser comes with two different heads: a cup-shaped head, which is good to use if you are sore, and a bullet-shaped head, for more concentrated therapy.

But, like all simulation devices, the Bio-Pulser is not perfect. It will help you beat the enemy to some degree, but it won't win the war. To correct muscle spasm, you must learn the manual stroking technique.

HOW *NOT* TO PERFORM A MASSAGE

Most forms of massage and physical therapy are palliative.

They temporarily relieve pain or tension by irritating the body and producing endorphins. They do not even begin to address what is really wrong.

When working with muscle—do *not*:

• Smash, grind, pummel, or rub the muscle.
• Massage the length of a muscle.
• Use long, heavy, slow pressure.
• Stretch the muscle or use traction.
• "Crack" or manipulate the vertebrae or joints.

These approaches all activate the stretch-reflex response.

Do *not*:

• Use heat, cold, ultrasound, or diathermy.

These are forms of thermal irritation.

And do *not*:

• Use sine-wave or any other type of electric current.

These are mild, but irritating forms of electrocution.

WHAT YOU MAY FEEL WHILE BEING MASSAGED

Sometimes my patients experience some pain or discomfort during treatment. Since I use relatively light pressure, what causes this? The more hypertonic the muscle is, the more it will hurt. The massage is not creating the pain—you are becoming aware of the pain that has been there all along but has been numbed by endorphins. It's a little like an alcoholic who finally stops drinking and has to face the feelings he has numbed with alcohol.

I've also heard rolfers claim that they are not causing the pain. The difference is, while I'm using a moderate fingertip pressure, they've got their elbows stuck into your muscle clear up to their biceps. *That* hurts!

SORENESS AFTER TREATMENT

At the beginning of a course of treatment, patients usually experience soreness after a massage. This is because a hard muscle is a sick muscle. As the spasm is relaxed, the lactic acid that has been stored in the muscle is released into the bloodstream, irritating the surrounding tissue. Histamine, which causes inflammation as part of the body's healing process, is also released.

PHYSIOLOGICAL CONTRACTURE

After you have relaxed all the outer layers of muscle, you get to the core spasm. This is a very different type of contraction from what we have discussed so far. It is called *physiological contracture* and has been described in Guyton's *Textbook of Medical Physiology* as living *rigor mortis*.

Most physiological contracture is actually the primordial spasm that developed when you were curled up in the uterus. It is completely locked up, so hard and contracted that it is not even capable of a stretch reflex. Releasing it, therefore, requires a different technique.

Physiological contracture feels almost like scar tissue and must be treated in the same way. You have to use heavy pressure to break through, but you cannot work on it until you have first released the outer layers of muscle from spasm. Because it is usually buried deeply, far away from any surrounding nerves, physiological contracture is almost never involved in nerve irritation, and most problems can be resolved without breaking it up. Nonetheless, if people are interested in achieving optimal health, they will want to have physiological contracture released.

HOW FREE OF SPASM CAN WE BECOME?

Our bodies are adaptive and inherently unstable organisms. For this reason, we will always be subject to a certain amount of spasticity just from the daily course of living. As you've seen, the condition of your muscles affects your health on many levels. So even after the spasm causing your symptoms has been released, it's a good idea to have periodic "tune-ups" to keep your muscles in good working order. You may feel fine, but remember, the body does not always communicate well with the brain. Most people do not become aware of disorders developing in their bodies until it's too late.

When clients ask me, "How many treatments do I need?" I say, "What do you want out of life?" If you want maximum health, this will be an ongoing process. I have some clients whose symptoms disappeared after a few months, but who have been with me for twenty-five years.

8
Exercise

here is so much misinformation about exercise, it would take another book to resolve all the confusion. Nevertheless, in this final chapter I would like to leave you with some information on exercises that are body-friendly.

One of the first things you learned way back in Chapter 2 was that the way most people exercise is unhealthy. So before we talk about body-friendly exercise, let's do a little recap of what you *don't* want to do and why.

EXERCISE DON'Ts

The following exercises make muscles spastic or aggravate existing ailments.

"Aerobic" Exercise

As you read in Chapter 2, the exercises we call "aerobic"—jogging, running, stair climbing, bicycling, using treadmills, and taking classes that push your heart rate up—are actually examples of *anaerobic* exercise. That is, they leave your muscles with an inadequate supply of oxygen, producing lactic acid and muscle spasm.

Popular exercise experts advise maintaining an exercise heart rate between 65 and 80 percent of maximum exertion for a minimum of twelve minutes. This is commonly thought to be an effective way to ensure true aerobic benefit from a workout. But the truth is, when your heart rate rises and you begin to pant for a sustained period of time, your muscles produce too much lactic acid. Although the exertion oxygenates the blood, it is not enough to prevent the high production of lactic acid. As a result, the muscles become spastic.

That's why joggers and other athletes often succumb to heart attacks. Exercise that increases your heart rate for extended periods of time is sheer trauma to the arterial muscles. An elevated heart rate is the result of increased levels of lactic acid in the bloodstream. This irritates the muscular walls of the coronary arteries, and can lead to arterial blockage, a major cause of heart attacks.

Bodybuilding

Bulging, defined, "cut" muscle is not healthy muscle. Lifting weights repetitively ensures that plenty of lactic acid gets trapped in the muscles, sickening the feedback nerves and causing permanent spastic contraction. You may look good, but sooner or later you'll stop feeling good.

Exercise For Back Problems

Some people think that exercising your abdominal muscles helps to strengthen your back. But this is physiologically impossible. The abdominals attach to the ribs and, for the most part, have no association with the muscles of the back. The only back muscle associated with abdominal movement is the psoas, but in bending your knees to perform most abdominal exercises, you totally avoid using the psoas.

It is also a mistake to advise people with back problems to perform repetitive exercises to strengthen the back muscles. Those problem back muscles are not really weak. They only seem weak because they are *overly* contracted. Exercises may relieve pain for a while, but they will only make the spasm worse. What should you do instead? That's like someone who's hitting himself in the head with a hammer asking what else he might do. Take a walk, have your muscles massaged according to the technique explained in Chapter 7. Just don't do those exercises.

Inactivity

Since your muscles work twenty-four hours a day to maintain tone, they always produce some lactic acid. Therefore, if you engage in little or no physical activity, your blood circulation becomes less efficient in flushing lactic acid from muscles. So if you lie around and do nothing, you're going to end up with spastic muscles.

THE LAST ANATOMY LESSON

You've got to exercise. But how? Before we talk about the most effective ways to work out, there's a little more muscle physiology you'll have to learn.

Fast-twitch and Slow-twitch Muscle

Every muscle is composed of two types of muscle fiber, fast-twitch and slow-twitch, which play an important role in understanding exercise and metabolism.

Only your slow-twitch muscle fibers can metabolize fatty acids. This is highly desirable for two reasons: Fat metabolism is always aerobic, burns cleanly, and does not produce lactic acid; in addition, it can draw directly on your stored body fat and help to reduce it.

Fast-twitch muscle fiber can only metabolize glucose.

During heavy exercise, some of this process will be aerobic, but most of it will be anaerobic and produce lactic acid.

The faster or more vigorous the exercise, the more you engage the fast-twitch fibers and leave the slow-twitch fibers behind—burning less fat and producing more lactic acid. Believe it or not, when you are at rest, your body is burning four times more fat than glucose. (But this doesn't mean you'll lose weight if you lie around and do nothing. We're talking *ratio* not quantity of fat burned.)

When I talk about moderate exercises that use slow-twitch fibers, many people think of marathon running. Are they ever wrong! On level ground you begin to leave the slow-twitch fibers behind at 8 or 9 miles an hour—but the average speed for a marathon runner is 11.5 miles an hour. That's why they stock up on carbohydrates before a race—it's the only fuel for fast-twitch muscles.

Some fitness experts claim that unless you are exercising so vigorously that you can't talk, you are burning fat. This is absolutely untrue. The changeover from fat to glucose happens gradually, from the moment you begin to move, and by the time you are doing "moderate" aerobics, you are burning no fat at all.

There's one more reason why fast vigorous exercise doesn't accomplish what it's supposed to. If you are using only fast-twitch fibers—you are using only *half* your muscle. The benefit of slow movement is that it uses both fast- and slow-twitch fibers, in other words, *all* of your muscle.

Endurance Versus Stamina

The low pulse rate that develops with vigorous exercise is not always a sign of fitness. To understand why, you must grasp the distinction between stamina and endurance.

When you have stamina, you have achieved a low pulse rate by increasing your muscle capillaries and strengthening your diaphragm.

When you exercise vigorously for sustained periods of

time, the low pulse rate you eventually achieve is only partly stamina. The rest is endurance, which means you are enduring—but not happily—lactic acid toxicity. Your liver has become *desensitized* to the level of lactic acid in your bloodstream and stops demanding enough oxygen to keep the level down. That's why your pulse rate slows. But lactic acid is still pouring through your bloodstream, as toxic as ever. That's why a trained athlete can take as long as an hour to recover from vigorous exercise, when it might take a neophyte only fifteen minutes.

Real fitness is stamina, not endurance. To achieve it your body must efficiently eliminate lactic acid from the muscles as you work out.

BODY-FRIENDLY EXERCISE

Summing up all we have learned so far, body-friendly exercise should:

- produce a minimum of lactic acid.
- increase circulation to help flush lactic acid out of the muscle.
- use all your muscle—both fast- and slow-twitch fibers.
- burn a greater proportion of fat than glucose.
- and build stamina rather than endurance.

Let's see what fits the bill.

Walking

Walking at a rate of about 3 miles an hour on level ground is one of the very best exercises you can do.

This pace allows your muscles to work with a minimum of anaerobically produced lactic acid. All of your muscle fibers, both the slow-twitch fat burners and the fast-twitch glucose burners are working. And the veins in your calves, which pump blood back up to the heart, have adequate time to fully refill between contractions. This promotes circulation and flushes your body clean. When you walk at this easy pace, blood moves through the body faster than needed to keep up with the lactic acid being produced.

Walking will burn calories much more cleanly than running, and you will be burning a higher ratio of fat to glucose.

The Best Way to Walk

The Europeans have a much better way of walking than we Americans do, and we could benefit from copying them.

We have a jaunty walk. We lift one leg, push it out ahead, the spring off from the balls and toes. This extra bounce puts unnecessary stress on your muscles—and going up and down instead of froward is wasted motion.

When you walk any distance at all, your feet get tired, because the metatarsal arch of your toes was not made to support so much weight. Not only that, but when you throw all your weight forward, your body tips backward for counterbalance, so it's almost like climbing uphill.

The bounce in your walk also blocks circulation, by causing prolonged tightening of the soleus muscles of the calf, restricting the flow of blood back up to your heart.

The Europeans plant their feet flat and push their bodies along in a walk that's driven by the heel, not the toes. This walk puts the larger muscle to work, helping circulation and minimizing lactic acid.

Here's how to do it. Let your trailing leg extend out far enough behind to feel a slight stretch in the calf muscle. Then lift your hip—not your thigh—slightly, and allow the leg to swing freely forward. The foot should land flat, with the weight evenly distributed between the heel and toes.

For most of us, walking is an unconscious habit, so it's a little awkward when you tamper with it. But with practice this walk can become second nature, and the benefits it brings will be well worth the effort.

Warming Up

Before doing any type of exercise, you should warm up your muscles by walking at a brisk pace (about $4^1/2$ miles an hour) for three to five minutes. It is not necessary to stretch before you exercise, but if you feel you must, do it as described below.

Stretching

Athletes used to stretch as a warm-up before exercise. Most now realize that it's not good to stretch cold muscle, yet still think that as long as you warm up first, it's fine to hold a stretch. It's not. Whether your muscles are warm or cold, holding a stretch causes a powerful reflex contraction. A stretch and hold exercise will temporarily lengthen the tendon, while shortening the muscle.

Stretching will benefit the muscles if you use the following technique to avoid turning on the stretch reflex. First, take a brisk warm-up walk. Then stretch to the point of strain—but do not pause there—and return to neutral posture in one smooth movement. You can repeat this as many times as you like. Your range will increase slightly with each repetition, up to a point. Don't make a heroic effort to pass that point. You may get a short-term result, but eventually you'll pay for it with even tighter muscles.

If you are attracted to Eastern forms of exercise, avoid yoga postures, because they involve prolonged stretching and holding. T'ai chi, with its slow, flowing movement, is a far better practice for the health of your body.

The Heavy/Light Principle

The heavy/light principle is a way of modifying many forms of exercise so that they will be beneficial. If you exercise with maximum exertion for a short period of time, slow down or relax for a few moments, then go full-tilt again, your body will have time to deal with the lactic acid being produced.

In an aerobics class, go all out for 3 minutes, walk for 5, then go all out again. With a stair-climber, stationary bike, or other machine that uses specific muscles intensely, work as hard as you can for one minute, then walk for two minutes. You can repeat this cycle as many times as you want.

The best kinds of sports call for intermittent, as opposed to constant, activity. Tennis, badminton, and squash are good. Racquetball and handball are far too fast because the harder ball moves at an extremely high velocity. (I've seen racquetball players in t-shirts that read "Harvey Wallbanger"—clearly describing another good reason these overly fast sports can be hard on your muscles.)

Wind Sprints

One of the very best ways to develop pure stamina is by doing wind sprints.

First, run as fast as you can for a block, then walk for two blocks so that the lactic acid can get flushed out of the muscles into the bloodstream. When it reaches the liver, it will be converted back into glucose, which will continue to fuel your muscles. You may sprint and walk like this for as long as you can.

You'll be developing stamina and expending energy, while at the same time keeping your muscles healthy.

Bicycling

Bicycling is wonderful exercise when you do it in a nice flat area. If you can coast a little, pedal a little, coast some more, you can ride for miles and it will be very beneficial for your body. Of course, the average bicycle seat can be pretty tough on the muscles it presses against, so use a gel seat. A recumbent bike is also excellent, because it allows you to sit on your gluteus maximus muscles, which are flat and can take the pressure.

Just remember, as soon as you begin panting, go light.

Training With Weights

Training properly with weights—as power lifters do—is an ideal exercise. But as soon as you say power lifter, people usually think of grossly obese men almost as fat as sumo wrestlers. Those are the heavyweight lifters, the 250 pound and over group, and they are one end of the spectrum.

But power lifters who weigh less than 250 pounds must stay slim, because the lower the weight class they make it into, the greater their advantage.

These power lifters have smooth, strong muscles. They do not have cut and definition the way bodybuilders do, and that's good, because as you know, that's hypertonic, spastic muscle.

When you power lift, work with as heavy a weight as you can—but take no more than six seconds to lift it once and set it down. This is because your muscles have a small store of oxygen that will last for just about six seconds. In order for the muscle to replenish its oxygen, you must rest for a full five seconds before you lift the weight again.

One slow lift for a full six seconds is far better than several repetitions in the same amount of time. First, the slow movement uses all your muscle fibers, whereas the faster repetitions use mostly the fast-twitch fibers. Second, slow movement burns fat, not just glucose.

After working one muscle group, walk around for two or three minutes before starting the next group.

Machines are better than free weights because you can completely let go after a heavy lift. With the exception of a bench press, where you can set the weight back on a holder, you can not let go of a free weight, so there is no pause that refreshes.

Power lifting builds healthy muscle, muscle that is

actually much stronger than the bound-up, bulked-out spasms you see on bodybuilders.

After You Exercise

Whenever you work out, take a walk afterward to help flush out the lactic acid. I'd also recommend taking a walk after athletic sex, but I don't think this practice will catch on soon.

How Often Should You Exercise?

You can walk every day. All other exercise should be done every other day at most.

Ideally, you should take a walk first thing in the morning to stimulate your circulation. When you wake up, you're in a polluted condition, because inactivity has slowed your blood flow, and lactic acid has been accumulating in your muscles all night. Do not do any other type of exercise when first awakening, because it will only add to the toxicity.

Hot Tubs and Showers

Extreme heat and ice cold showers will drive your muscles into spasm, but here's what you can do to relax.

It's perfectly fine to sit in a tub that's no hotter than 96 degrees. Have all the swirling, bubbling water you like—but no jets pounding into your muscles, making them tighten up.

A pulsating shower massager is good, because the water does not come out in a steady stream but pulses. If it's not too hot and not too hard, this can be very relaxing for your muscles.

So there it is. You can and should keep on exercising. Just modify what you do, and you'll not only look good, and feel good, you'll be genuinely improving your health.

Conclusion

This book is a beginning. The information you've just absorbed should give you a better understanding of what is really going on in your body and help you to find real health and healing.

I hope that this work will also stimulate the medical community to become interested in the vitally important area of muscle physiology. It would be a great step forward if doctors and other practitioners could begin to understand how muscle dysfunction—not just the structural reaction to this dysfunction—is the genesis of many ailments that do not respond to current methods of treatment. At the very least, perhaps we could see an end to the prescription of harmful and unnecessary surgery and medication.

As for me, many mysteries remain. I am still observing and learning the complexities of muscle; my understanding and knowledge of it are still developing. This work is not something completed or perfected. It is work in progress.

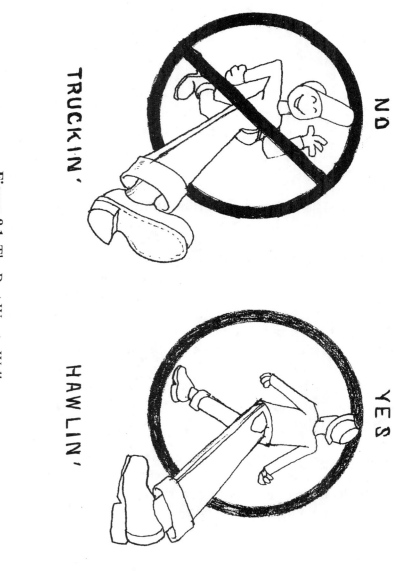

Figure 8.1 The Best Way to Walk

Bibliography

Grant, J.C. Boileau, *Grant's Atlas of Anatomy*. 6th Edition
Baltimore: The Williams and Walkins Co., 1972

Han, Man-Chung and Kim, Cau-Wan *Sectional Human Anatomy*.
Second Printing, New York: Igaku-Shoin, 1985

Mountcastle, Vernon, *Medical Physiology*. Thirteenth Edition
St. Louis: C.V. Mosby Co., 1974

Schmidt, R. F., *Fundamentals of Neurophysiology*. Third Edition
New York: Springer-Verlag, 1985

Guyton, Arthur C. *Textbook of Medical Physiology*. 3rd ed.
Philadelphia: W. B. Saunders Company, 1966.

Williams, Warwick, Dyson, and Bannister, eds. *Gray's Anatomy*.
37th ed. London: Churchill and Livingstone, 1989

Index

Morphine, 56
Moxibustion, 32
MRI. *See* Magnetic reso-
nance imaging.
MS. *See* Multiple sclerosis,
120
Multifidus to the third
lumbar vertebra, 65,
66, 67, 76, 77, 100
Multiple sclerosis (MS),
120, 121
Muscle, 45
attitudes toward, 43
cardiac, 45
smooth, 46
skeletal, 46–47
Muscle, skeletal, 41
flat, 46–47, 48, 49
round, 46, 47, 48
Muscle, smooth, 41
Muscle atrophy, 18
Muscle fibers
bag, 52, 53
chain, 52, 53
fast-twitch (white), 46,
54, 155–156
slow-twitch (dark), 46,
155–156
Muscle reserve, 57–58
Muscle spasm, 8–9, 25, 43,
44–45, 55–56, 58–60
healing, 141–152
pattern of, 63–94, 134,
144
Muscle spindle, 51–53
Muscle tone, 47, 49–50
Myelin, 120

Mysticism, 35

Nearsightedness, 116–117
Neck
crick in the, 71
stiff, 72–73
Nerve stress, 59–60
Nerve summation, 71
Neuroendocrine glands,
40
Neuroendocrine system,
108
Non-neuroendocrine
glands, 40

Oblique, external, 117, 135,
136
Obliquus capitis inferior,
109
Obliquus capitis superior,
109, 115
Obturator internus, 113,
137
Occipital nerve, greater,
108, 109, 116
Occipital nerve, lesser, 109,
115, 116
Occipital nerve, third, 109,
116
Orinase, 124
Orthokeratology, 117
Orthopedic stress, 60
Osteoarthritis, 94–95
Osteoblast, 126
Osteoclast, 126
Osteoporosis, 126–127
Ovaries, 121